I0845433

Menopause Mentor

Your Guide Through Menopause

Rebecca Hellbusch, RN

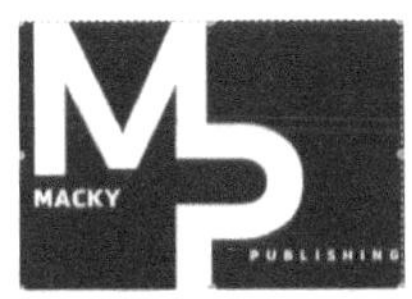

Contents

Your Guide
Through Menopause

To my Sisters in Menopause, You've got this
Cheers

Rebecca Hellbusch, RN

© Copyright 2023 - Rebecca Hellbusch All rights reserved.

It is not legal to reproduce, duplicate, or transmit any part of this document in either electronic means or in printed format. Recording this publication is strictly prohibited, and any storage of this document is not allowed unless with written permission from the publisher, except for using brief quotations in a book review.

This book is a work of nonfiction. Any resemblance to persons, living or dead, or places, events, or locations is purely coincidental.

All rights reserved. This book or any portion thereof may not be reproduced or used in any manner whatsoever without the publisher's express written permission except for the use of brief quotations in a book review.

Cover Design by _________

Illustrations by (if applicable) _______

Printed in _______ (country or platform)

First edition, 2022. www.MarkyPublishing.com

Introduction

Shh! Listen. Did you hear that?

No, it wasn't the wind or the hum of a motor.

It's the collective sigh of millions of exasperated middle-aged women as they realize they are about to experience a change. It's menopause!

No, it's not enough that they have endured years, decades even, of monthly inconvenience and sometimes downright pain and discomfort. Their lady parts have successfully been churning out eggs to ensure the continuation of the human race. But, whether they birthed children or not, the menstrual cycle has often been a very bumpy, uncomfortable trip.

But now the ovaries are beginning to slow down, and notice has been given. It's time for this chapter in their lives to end. But menstruation will not go quietly. Oh, no! That would be too simple. From all accounts, this transition could be just as stormy!

But ladies, I know you. No, not personally. But I know women. You are strong and resilient and will come out on the other side of menopause triumphant, joyful, and ready to enjoy your midlife to the fullest.

If only you knew about the misinformation and the lack of information about the menopausal transition and menopause itself, you'd be shocked and maybe even angry. Without facts, managing the multitude of symptoms that the menopause transition brings is like assembling a desk from Ikea without the instruction manual. You might get close but find out later that you placed a drawer in backward, and the damn desk doesn't work as it should.

Sister, I want you to function at 100% during your transition and after menopause is complete. But to do that, you need the facts! Then, equipped and armed with knowledge, you'll face any fear and conquer your worry about:

- Hot flashes. *I'm worried I'll sweat through my clothes at work. How embarrassing!*
- Night sweats. *Sleep is as essential as air to me. I require a good night's rest-every night!*
- Lagging sex drive. *I love sex! My partner loves sex. I don't want this to stop!*
- Mood swings. *Mood swings before and during my period were terrible. So what's going to happen now?*

- Joint and muscle pain. *Another day and I'm waking up with a new ache. Will this ever stop?*
- Irregular periods. *I just had a period two weeks ago. What the hell?*

My experience is that you can conquer anxiety, worry, and fear when you face your challenges head-on. Imagine having a plan and actions you can take to control and manage any symptom that impacts your quality of life during your transition into menopause and beyond.

Breathe easy. It's all right here.

I'll provide nightly steps, a routine you can implement that improves your sleep health.

Are you worried about managing hot flashes at work or while on the town? You'll learn common-sense tips to keep you cool and all about avoiding environmental triggers.

I'll walk you through step-by-step each stage of menopause, what to expect, the good, the bad, and the ugly.

And you'll hear about all the medical and alternative treatment options available to you so that you can make the best health decisions.

I have prepared this book to empower you with knowledge so you can navigate menopause gracefully and confidently and live life to the fullest!

I am a healthcare professional with 25 years of experience as a registered nurse. I am passionate about advocating for women's health during this time. I believe women should feel confident and informed so they can take charge of their health decisions and know that each choice they make benefits them and that they're not just a name and number on a chart.

Ladies, I am honored to walk with you on your health journey through menopause. Let's begin.

Chapter 1

PeriMenopause

"Gravity and wrinkles are fine with me. They're a small price to pay for the new wisdom inside my head and heart." ~ *Drew Barrymore*

That time has arrived that you have heard about since you started your first period. It is the time in your life when Aunt Flo, as my mother used to call it, stops coming around as much. You are not quite as worried about shopping and being caught unaware because that time of the month showed up two days early. And we don't even need to talk about the messes and stained clothing.

So, while there are a lot of advantages to this time in your life, there will be a lot of questions – maybe even some fear or anxiety. That's normal, and that is why I'm here to help.

Let's start talking about perimenopause and what you can expect from this time in your life.

Perimenopause means around menopause. This is also known as the menopausal transition. It is a natural change in your life. Women enter into menopause at different ages. Some women might start seeing changes in their bodies as early as their thirties, such as irregular periods. Other women might notice changes once they are in their forties (Mayo Clinic, 2023).

Perimenopause normally drops in on us in our mid-forties to mid-fifties. The National Institute on Aging (NIA) states menopause usually lasts around seven years but can last up to fourteen years. Many factors can affect how long menopause lasts, such as smoking, ethnicity, and the age at which it begins.

Perimenopause occurs because your estrogen levels rise and fall. Estrogen is the main female hormone and is mostly made in your ovaries. These hormones are responsible for many things, such as regulating your menstrual cycle, heart and blood vessels, the brain, pelvic muscles, skin, hair, breasts, etc. They also affect your urinary tract, reproductive tract, musculoskeletal, and cardiovascular systems (John Hopkins Health, 2023).

When your body is shifting toward perimenopause and the levels of estrogen rise and fall, you will start to notice changes. Your period might last longer than usual or be shorter than expected. Your body might not release an egg during some of the menstrual cycles. You may also start to experience other symptoms, such as vaginal dryness, insomnia, and, what I liked to call, my personal hell … hot flashes (Mayo Clinic, 2023). I

You will likely notice other changes during perimenopause. According to NIA (2023), your body will start to use its energy differently. As a result, your fat cells will change, and it is easier to gain weight. You might notice that your body changes shape and composition. In addition, you might experience changes in the health of your heart and bones. Your physical functions may also change.

Perimenopause ends, and menopause begins when you have gone twelve months without menstruation. We will talk about that in the next chapter.

Symptoms

The Mayo Clinic (2023) describes and explains the most common symptoms associated with perimenopause.

Irregular menstruation

The changes in menstruation were a little surprising to me. I had always thought they would slowly taper off until there were no more periods. I was in for a shock. Your periods may last longer, or they might be shorter. The flow can change as well. You might have a heavy flow one month and a very light flow the next. According to the Mayo Clinic (2023), if you have persistent changes in your period of seven days or more, it could signal that you are in early perimenopause. However, if the time between your periods is two months or more, that could indicate that you are in late perimenopause.

Hot flashes

My favorite – not. For me, the hot flashes felt like I was baking in a five thousand degrees oven, and I was afraid that I would experience spontaneous combustion. Luckily, that hasn't happened yet. However, your hot flashes will likely be different because the frequency, length, and intensity of the flashes differ for each woman.

NIA (2023) states that when you experience a hot flash, you might experience a sudden feeling of heat in the upper part of your body or over your entire body. You might be flushed in your face and neck. You could also see red splotches pop up on your chest, arms, and back. If that wasn't enough fun, you might experience heavy sweating and cold chills.

Sometimes the heat flashes are not that severe. However, some might be strong enough to wake you out of deep sleep. These are called night sweats. They usually last between thirty seconds to ten minutes. They can happen a couple of times an hour, a day, or just a few times a week (NIA, 2023). I have woken up with the sheets soaking wet. I was so tired I changed my t-shirt and put a towel down, and called it a night.

Sleeping problems

I have noticed that insomnia has befriended me. Perimenopause can cause you to have sleeping problems. One reason might be that it is hard to sleep when you are drenched in a pool of your own sweat when you have a hot flash. However, the Mayo Clinic (2023) says you might have difficulty sleeping simply because you have entered perimenopause.

Mood changes

My husband really enjoys this particular symptom of perimenopause. He loves it so much that he will invent chores outside of the house because he never knows whether he will have a run-in with Dr. Jekyll or Mrs. Hyde. While my mood could swing from happy to sad to angry in almost a split second, that might not be the same for you. Just like all the other symptoms, every person experiences mood swings differently.

As well as the abrupt mood changes, you might feel more irritable or even start suffering from depression. Some of these symptoms might be because you are experiencing insomnia, not getting restful sleep or the hot flashes you get. The Mayo Clinic (2023) says that your mood swings might not be linked to the hormonal changes perimenopause causes. So look at all your symptoms, and don't assume menopause equals antidepressants. Women often go to their physicians and are put on antidepressants because that's an easy answer in the doctors' eyes.

Vaginal and bladder issues

According to the Mayo Clinic (2023), intercourse might become painful during this period because the vaginal tissues might lose lubrication and aren't as elastic. The decrease in estrogen can also cause you to be more vulnerable to vaginal infections or urinary tract infections. The loss of tissue tone can also cause urinary incontinence. This was by far the worst symptom I experienced. Hopefully, you won't have to deal with it. But, if you do, there is a solution. I'll talk about that later.

A decrease in fertility

Because you are ovulating less frequently, your ability to have a child also decreases. However, you can still have a child, so unless you are ready for that, you should take precautions until you have gone a full twelve months without a period.

Changes in your sexual function

During perimenopause, your sexual arousal, and desire may change. However, the Mayo Clinic (2023) states that if your sex life was satisfying before your perimenopausal state, it would likely continue being satisfactory.

Bone loss

Decreases in estrogen levels can affect your bones. You will start to lose more bone than you will replace. This increases your risk of osteoporosis, which is a disease that causes your bones to be fragile. One of the best things you can do to keep your bones strong is to lift weights and keep moving.

Cholesterol level may change

The decrease in estrogen levels may lead to an unfortunate change in your cholesterol levels. You may see an increase in low-density lipoprotein (LDL) cholesterol, which is known as the bad cholesterol. This can increase your risk of heart disease. The loss of good cholesterol also contributes to an increase in heart disease. Your high-density lipoprotein (HDL), known as the good cholesterol, may decrease.

John Hopkins Medicine (2023) states additional symptoms you might experience when perimenopause sets in. These include headaches, trouble concentrating, joint and muscle aches, heavy sweating, needing to urinate more often, and having symptoms similar to PMS.

Early Onset of Perimenopause

Sometimes, women experience perimenopause earlier in their lives. Research suggests that there may be certain risk factors associated with this. These include smoking, family history, cancer treatments, and a hysterectomy. The Mayo Clinic (2023) states that when you just have your uterus removed, that process does not start perimenopause. You still ovulate; you just don't have periods. However, you might start the process sooner than average. In addition, you may experience early onset of perimenopause if one of your ovaries is removed, which can cause the second one to stop working sooner.

How Is Perimenopause Diagnosed?

Because the symptoms seem to sneak up on you and pounce when you aren't looking, it can be difficult to diagnose perimenopause. However, the doctor can look at your medical history, age, and symptoms and then conduct a physical exam as part of a diagnosis. In addition, you might have blood tests that can determine your estrogen levels.

When You Should See a Doctor

Not all women will see a doctor as soon as the symptoms

of perimenopause emerge. They can tolerate the symptoms without assistance, or their symptoms are not severe. The Mayo Clinic stated that because the symptoms are not always obvious and they appear gradually, you might not even notice them. If you do, you may not realize that they are all related to the same thing: the onset of perimenopause.

However, if your symptoms start interfering with your life or well-being, you should consider seeing a doctor. If your symptoms cause concern, you should also contact your doctor.

The Mayo Clinic (2023) suggests that you see a doctor if you start bleeding exceedingly heavily and are changing your pad or tampon every couple of hours. You should also visit your doctor if you bleed for more than seven days. In addition, you should consult with your physician if you bleed between your periods or if your regular periods are less than twenty-one days apart.

The Mayo Clinic (2023) says that there are several ways that you can prepare for your visit.

1. Record the last three months of your menstrual cycle. It should include the dates when your period began and when it ended. You should also note whether your period was heavy, medium, or light.

2. Create a list of any symptoms that you have experienced. You should include even the smallest details about your symptoms, such as how often you have hot flashes.

Ensure you include symptoms you don't think are related to perimenopause.

3. Write down any stress or life changes you have experienced lately.

4. Create a list of all the medications and supplements that you are taking. Make sure that you include how much the dosage is and when you take the medication.

5. Make a list of questions you want to ask the doctor. I know I always tell myself that I will remember to ask my doctor important questions but forget them during my appointment.

Treating Perimenopause

Unless your symptoms are severe, you will not normally need to be treated for perimenopause. However, the doctor might suggest some treatments if necessary.

Hormone therapy

According to the Mayo Clinic (2030) your doctor might prescribe hormone therapy that uses estrogen alone or estrogen along with progestins to help level out your hormone levels. These treatments may come in many different forms, such as a gel, patch, spray, or cream. Estrogen therapy is the most effective therapy for treating night sweats and hot flashes. The dose will depend on your and your family's medical history. Estrogen hormone treatment can also help with bone loss. If you still have your uterus, the doctor may also prescribe progestin.

. . .

Vaginal estrogen

The doctor can prescribe vaginal estrogen that can be applied straight to the vagina with a ring, tablet, or cream. Whichever the method, a minuscule amount of estrogen is released to be absorbed by the tissues in the vagina. The purpose is to help alleviate vaginal dryness and relieve discomfort during sex. It also relieves some urinary symptoms (Mayo Clinic, 2023).

Antidepressants

The doctor might also prescribe antidepressants or mood stabilizers to help with mood swings. Certain antidepressants, specifically selective serotonin reuptake inhibitors (SSRI) can help decrease the frequency and intensity of hot flashes. This method is ideal for women who cannot take estrogen or are already on antidepressants because they have a mood disorder.

Gabapentin or neurontin

Gabapentin is normally used to treat seizures but can also help decrease hot flashes. This therapy method is especially beneficial for women who cannot take estrogen or suffer from migraines.

Your doctor might also suggest exercising regularly and eating a healthy diet. Your diet should provide you with one thousand to two thousand milligrams of calcium daily through food or supplements. You can also keep a journal and take note of what causes your hot flashes, such as alcohol, tea, or coffee, so that you can avoid them (John Hopkins Medicine (2023).

Taking Care of Yourself During Perimenopause

Like it or not, being in the perimenopause state in your life may mean making some lifestyle changes that can be hard at first. Still, if you take it one day at a time, you can make the changes so that this part of your life is much less uncomfortable.

Mitigate vaginal discomfort

There are many water-based products you can purchase over the counter to help ease vaginal dryness. Astroglide and K-Y Jelly are lubricants that you can use to help sex be more enjoyable. Some moisturizers can reduce vaginal dryness, such as Replens or Vagisil Prohydrate. The Mayo Clinic (2023) states that you should choose products free from glycerin, as that ingredient could cause a burning sensation or irritation if you are sensitive to it. If you are sexually active, that will also help relieve vaginal dryness or discomfort because it increases the blood flow to that area.

Healthy eating

The Mayo Clinic (2023) states that because of risk of osteoporosis and heart disease increases during this time, you must eat healthily. You should eat a low-fat diet that is high in fiber. You need to be eating a lot of fruits and vegetables, as well as whole grains and food that are calcium-rich. As much as you might need that glass of wine after dinner or that cup of coffee to get your motor running in the morning, you may have to cut them out of your diet if they contribute to your heart flashes. You should talk to your doctor about whether you need to take calcium as a supplement. Your doctor will advise you on what supplements to take and how much you need daily. If the doctor recommends a calcium supplement, you should ask whether you should also take a vitamin D supplement, as it helps with calcium absorption.

Stay active

As with eating healthy, staying active is important for almost every health condition and issue. Although you might be tired of having people tell you to stay active, it is crucial as you go through the perimenopause state of your life. As the Mayo Clinic (2023) reports, exercising regularly can help prevent weight gain, which is an issue with perimenopause. It will also help you sleep better at night and will help elevate your mood. In addition, research indicates that including an exercise regimen in your life on a regular basis can decrease the risk of hip fractures in older women and strengthen bone density. You should exercise for at least half an hour almost every day, although not right before you hit the hay.

Hahns Petty, an exercise physiologist at the Piedmont Atlanta Fitness Center, states that exercising regularly can help you balance your hormones naturally (Piedmont, 2023). There are several hormones that are affected by exercise (Piedmont, 2023):

1. Dopamine: Dopamine is a hormone that your brain produces. It helps to reduce stress levels and can help mitigate the symptoms of depression. Dopamine is referred to as runners' high because it helps enhance the transmitters

responsible for positive feelings. Dopamine also helps decrease the anxious feeling associated with stress.

2. Serotonin: Exercise helps with the brain's serotonin production, known as the feel-good hormone. It can encourage positive moods, a good night's rest, memory, sexual function, appetite, and digestion.

3. Testosterone: Believe it or not, women also produce and use testosterone. While too much of anything is never good, you need the right testosterone levels to be healthy.

4. Estrogen: Exercising so your heart rate increases at least half an hour daily can help increase estrogen production and decrease the negative symptoms associated with perimenopause.

Get enough rest

I know -- this is much easier said than done. Between night sweats and insomnia, this just isn't always feasible. In chapter five, we will discuss foods that can help you sleep. Try not to partake in caffeine within a few hours before you go to bed. And even though that glass of wine or beer sounds great and relaxing, alcohol can interrupt your sleep.

Use stress reduction techniques

As you know, stress will only exacerbate any negative symptoms of perimenopause. My husband tells me to stop stressing out, but unfortunately, that doesn't help. I have no magic spell that makes it go away. However, there are ways that you can reduce the stress in your life. Meditation, yoga, and breathing exercises can help you relax and reduce your stress. We will talk about different types of meditation, yoga poses, and other relaxation methods in Chapter Six.

Alternative medicine

There are also several alternative medicines you can take to replace or complement conventional medicine. This will be discussed in Chapter Five.

Conclusion

Perimenopause happens around the time of your period. It is a life change that usually occurs in women in their thirties or forties. However, it can appear sooner or later than that.

Symptoms subtly and gradually appear, so you may not even know you are experiencing them. You might not even know that you have arrived at this change in your life because the symptoms are not always so obvious initially.

Although some of the symptoms are unpleasant to deal with, there are many ways to manage them. You should start by contacting your doctor to discuss your symptoms and what treatments are available that can help you find relief. Make sure you write down a list of questions you have, any medications you might be taking, and a list of your symptoms and the severity of each.

Have you made that phone call to set up your appointment? Great. Now, stand up, stretch, and get something to drink as we move into the next chapter – menopause.

Chapter 2

Menopause

"You can do this - this thing, where your body will cease to produce hormones and your skin, hair, muscles and bones ... basically every part of you will notice, go into withdrawals, and stage a coup. Be prepared for this mentally, and you'll own this 'thing'."
~ Lisa Key Davis, author

Perimenopause has led you to your next journey in life – menopause. It is a natural transition as your body ages. You are considered to have entered menopause when you have gone twelve straight months without having experienced a period.

Sometimes, this can be a challenging part of your life because there are other changes in your life, as well. For example, you might be tasked with helping out with your aging parents, and your children might finally be moving out to start their own lives. You might even be experiencing career changes.

You might have a hot flash while taking your parent to a doctor's appointment and another while making dinner. It is bad enough that you think your radiant heat is cooking the meal instead of the stove. Then, out of the blue, you stop singing along with your favorite song and shoot daggers at the world because you are so irritable.

Oh, wait – that's me.

One of the most important things to remember when thinking about menopause is that no two women will experience it the same way. Your mother may have experienced it one way, you another, and your best friend still another way.

For some, menopause is a relief. You don't have to worry about your period coming to wreak havoc in your life – not to mention all the money you will save by not purchasing feminine hygiene products. For others, it is a relief that there won't be any more last-minute babies sneaking in, so you are in your seventies when they graduate from high school. Fifty-six was bad enough!

Symptoms

While there might be these perks, there might also be some negative aspects to menopause. As your estrogen levels continue to decrease, you will notice even more changes in your body. Of course, the symptoms associated with peri-menopause will still be present and will be less severe for some than they are for others. Some women won't be bothered; some will suffer from hot flashes, insomnia, painful sex, mood swings, and depression.

Hot flashes

You may continue to enjoy hot flashes during menopause and even after it ends. Exciting news, right?

However, NIA (2023) states that there are treatments that can help reduce the severity of your hot flashes. It is important that you create a journal of your hot flashes, including what you are eating or doing before they happen. That way, you can have an idea of what triggers them.

Lifestyle changes can have a tremendous impact on your hot flashes and their severity, according to NIA (2023).

1. Wear layered clothes that you can remove when the hot flash starts.

2. Carry a portable fan.

3. Avoid alcohol, caffeine, and spicy foods.

4. If you smoke, try to quit.

5. Try to maintain a healthy weight, as overweight and obese women tend to experience more hot flashes.

6. Explore mind and body exercises. (We will talk about some of these in Chapter Six.)

Your doctor may also prescribe some nonhormonal medication for you. One of those medications is paroxetine, which is an SSRI (described in Chapter One). If you are prescribed this or an antidepressant to treat hot flashes, then you will take a lower dose than women taking them for mental health disorders (NIA 2023).

Hormone therapy is another choice that you and your

doctor might decide on. It can level the amounts of estrogen and progesterone in your body. This decision must be discussed very carefully with your doctor because it has been known to increase your risk of breast cancer, gallbladder disease, heart attack, stroke, blood clots, and dementia (NIA, 2023). I know this sounds like a lot, but you can and will handle it. I believe every woman needs to weigh the pros and cons of HRT and include quality of life in that equation. For me, supplementing estrogen was the only way I could have sex without being in pain and bleeding. My doctor told me I would be at risk, albeit very small, with some of the complications mentioned above. I decided it's a risk I accepted to have that physical connection with my spouse. It's your body and your choice. You will have to decide what is best for you. Just know there are solutions, but some come with risks.

Bladder control

Have you ever sneezed and suddenly felt the dread of that trickle, and you just knew that you had a wee bit of an accident? I have, and it's a little bit embarrassing. You might also have a sudden urge to urinate or experience leaking. This is referred to as incontinence. You should see your doctor if this occurs. There are some medications that you can go on that will help. You can also use pads or adult diapers.

Urinary tract infections

Unfortunately, you may also have an increase in urinary tract infections during menopause. It is usually a bladder infection. One symptom is that you feel a burning sensation when you urinate. These are usually caused by bacteria from the bowel getting into the bladder or urethra. Your doctor will ask you to pee in a cup, review your family history, and conduct an exam to determine whether you have a urinary tract infection. Treatment usually consists of taking an antibiotic and drinking a lot of water or other liquids to flush your system. You can help prevent these by drinking plenty of fluids and practicing good hygiene (National Institute of Diabetes…, 2023). A helpful suggestion to prevent a UTI is always peeing after sex.

Sleep problems

Sweet Morpheus, Greek God of ever-elusive sleep, has forgotten you – again. You either can't get to sleep or stay asleep, or you wake up way too early. Unfortunately, this is something that women who are going through menopause experience. Night sweats may also be the culprit (NIA, 2023). We will discuss ways to help you get a better night's sleep in Chapter Five

Vaginal health and sexuality

As you know, either from the previous chapter or by experience, vaginal dryness is one of the annoying symptoms of menopause. You might also experience itching, burning, and a tightening of the vaginal opening. That is not only uncomfortable, but it can make sex painful. You can talk to your doctor about these issues. The doc can suggest different remedies on how to alleviate the symptoms, such as vaginal cream (NIA, 2023).

If you experience painful sex, you might consider using water-soluble lubricants. You can also try vaginal moisturizers that you can buy over the counter. These are used regularly and not just while you are having intercourse. The doctor might also prescribe hormones that will help with the problem. Like an estrogen patch. They might also prescribe either ospemifene or prasterone, which are non-hormone treatment options.

Changes in your mood

My husband and children *love* my mood swings. When I'm feeling good and peppy, my daughter loves to go shopping with me, because she can usually talk me into buying her things that she really doesn't need. Then, there are the times when they cross their fingers and yell, "Begone Demon," before they run for cover.

According to the NIA (2023), researchers are not entirely sure why women in menopause suffer from mood swings, depression, and irritability. It may be linked to other stress, like caring for aging parents, supporting (not necessarily money-wise) your adult children, or simple fatigue. If you are experiencing these types of mood swings, depression, anxiety, or just stress, then you should talk to your doctor. Your doctor may prescribe antidepressants or mood stabilizers to help you through these feelings.

Your body feels different

When I was younger, I was cute. I had a decent body and I turned more than one head. Now that I am going through menopause, I hate to look in the mirror. I am no longer that well-built cutie that used to stroll through the mall or the grocery store.

The fact is, that during this transition time, your body will change. Your waist, like mine, may grow. You might not be as muscular and have gained more fat. Your skin might become very thin (NIA, 2023). Right now, all I have to do is look at my skin, and it bleeds.

If that isn't enough, you might notice that your joints, muscles, and even your body start to feel stiff and ache. You might begin to have headaches and heart palpitations. Talk to a doctor if you begin to experience any of these symptoms.

Concentration and memory

You might have noticed your memory is slipping slightly (NIA, 2023). I can walk into a room, fully intent on something, and then forget why I am there. Let's not even talk about what happens when I try to put something in a safe place and then don't remember where I put it. It stays safe, especially from me. It is important to call your doctor if you're having issues with your memory.

Research shows that there are ways that you can help stimulate your brain and help to prevent memory loss (Cleveland Health Clinic, 2023), such as:

1. Crossword puzzles, math problems, reading, and other activities that will stimulate your brain.

2. Exercise.

3. Reducing passive activities, such as watching television.

Other symptoms

Although the above symptoms are the most common, there are others that you might experience due to being in menopause, as mentioned by Cleveland Health Clinic (2023):

1. Dry skin, eyes, or mouth

2. More sensitive teeth and gums, and an increase in developing gingivitis and cavities

3. Tender breasts

4. Changes in your sex drive

5. Difficulty concentrating

6. Hair thinning or hair loss

7. Increase in facial hair due to a decrease in estrogen and an increase in testosterone

8. Aggressiveness

9. Anxiety and stress

10. A lack of motivation

We will discuss how to motivate yourself, ways to address anxiety and stress, as well as ways to improve concentration and focus in Chapter Five.

Long-term effects

A lot of these symptoms will disappear over time. However, some long-term effects are more serious – osteoporosis and coronary artery disease.

Osteoporosis

Osteoporosis, also called brittle bone disease, happens when the inside of your bones becomes less dense. This makes them fragile and easier to break. Estrogen helps to preserve your bone mass and sends signals to your bones to stop breaking down.

According to the Cleveland Health Clinic (2023), due to a loss of estrogen, an average of women lose twenty-five percent of their bone mass from menopause until they are sixty. This contributes to bone fractures.

Cleveland Health Clinic (2023) states that your doctor will want to test your bone strength. Bone mineral testing, which is also referred to as bone densitometry, can help determine how much calcium is in certain parts of your bones. The bone density test, DEXA, uses low levels of ex-rays to see how dense your bones are and whether you are suffering from osteopenia (the precursor to osteoporosis) or osteoporosis. If it is found that you do suffer from low bone density or one of the other diseases, then your doctor may prescribe estrogen to treat it.

Coronary heart disease

Cleveland Health Clinic (2023) states that, unfortunately, menopause can also cause coronary heart disease. This is when arteries that supply blood to your heart either narrow or are blocked because fatty plaque builds up in the artery walls, referred to as atherosclerosis. High levels of choles-terol in your blood often cause atherosclerosis. Once menopause has moved in, your chances of this increase for several reasons:

1. Decrease in estrogen levels
2. Increased blood pressure
3. Decrease in physical activity

4. Specific lifestyle habits, such as smoking or excessive drinking of alcohol

Whether or not hormone replacement therapy can help prevent these long-term effects of menopause depends on your age and your health. Cleveland Health Clinic (2023) states that younger women tend to benefit more than those who are postmenopausal or are in their sixties.

Seek Medical Attention

I know you are strong, and medical care is expensive. However, there are some times during your menopausal journey when you need to seek out medical help to ensure that you stay healthy, such as:

Bleeding after menopause

If you bleed vaginally after intercourse, it normally isn't anything to be worried about. As mentioned, vaginal dryness is one of the many symptoms of perimenopause and menopause. This means that your vaginal tissues can become irritated during intercourse.

However, if you start bleeding vaginally and there is no good reason for it, then you need to contact your doctor as soon as possible. You also need to see your doctor if you have a foul-smelling or other type of discharge. This could be a sign of uterine cancer. Your doctor will likely want to conduct some tests (Gennev, 2023).

Fractures before menopause

If you have suffered bone fractures after age fifty, but before you enter menopause, you must see a doctor. These factors can indicate that you are at a higher risk of osteoporosis. If the bone density tests indicate that you do not suffer from this condition, you and your doctor can find a way to mitigate any future risk (Gennev, 2023).

Autoimmune or thyroid issues

If you have many of the signs of menopause, such as brain fog, weight gain, hot flashes, etc., and you suffer from an autoimmune disease or you, or anyone in your family, have thyroid issues, you should go see your doctor (Gennev, 2023).

Excessive sweating

As you know, night sweats are a symptom of menopause. However, if you suffer from excessive sweating, it may be time to see the doctor because it might be a sign of a serious illness or disease, such as a heart attack or lymphoma. Gennev (2023) states that if you happen to be "sweating through the bed sheets" every night, and you also seem to be experiencing other symptoms, such as rapid weight gain or loss, or a lump in your neck, throat, armpit, or groin, then you need to go visit a doctor.

Cognitive brain issues

It's one thing to forget where you've put your keys every once in a while or forget why you walked into a room. However, if you are having difficulty keeping up with a conversation, forget what month or year it is, how old you are, or forget to pay your bills, then it is time to go to the doctor. Also, if your friends and family start to notice changes in your personality, you should see a doctor. These could be symptoms of a more serious disease, such as dementia or Alzheimer's (Gennev, 2023).

Headaches

If you are prone to headaches, then they tend to decrease after forty. However, if you have an increase in the number of headaches that you have after menopause, then that could be a sign of something more serious. If your headaches are accompanied by a myriad of other symptoms, such as chills, fevers, muscle aches, nausea, or weight loss, then you should contact your doctor. In addition, if the headaches get worse when you stand up, or they get progressively worse, you should contact your doctor. However, Gennev (2023) states that you shouldn't let regular headaches cause you stress, because tension headaches and migraines are common forms of headaches during this time in your life.

Back pain

There are many causes of back pain, such as sitting too much, your mattress, and bad posture. However, Gennev (2023) states that you need to check the back pain out if it is localized. This is especially true if you have osteoporosis or a family history of cancer. If your pain worsens during the night when you are in bed or taking deep breaths, or it happens without you doing any strenuous activity, then you should talk to your doctor. It is even more important to talk to your doctor if the back pain is accompanied by fatigue, unexplained weight loss, or a cough – especially if you are coughing up blood. Gennev (2023) states that approximately twenty-five percent of people with lung cancer said they had upper to middle back pain before being diagnosed.

In addition, lower back pain accompanied by constipation, pelvic pain, bloating, urinary tract issues, or a loss of appetite should be immediately reported to the doctor. These symptoms could indicate ovarian cancer (Gennev, 2023).

Conclusion

There are a lot of similarities in what you will experience during your perimenopause menopausal stage of life. The symptoms and treatments are similar.

You must monitor your health during menopause, and if something doesn't seem right, especially if your symptoms seem more extreme than normal, make sure you contact your doctor. Don't forget to take notes on your symptoms and a list of questions you might have.

As a matter of fact, grab your computer or a notebook and do that now. What symptoms have you been experiencing? How intense are they? What questions do you have for your doctor?

Are you finished? Excellent. Let's talk about late menopause and what you need to know if you experience menopause after you turn fifty-five. Then, we will talk about hormone replacement therapy so that you can decide whether it might be right for you.

Chapter 3

Late Menopause

"The changes, the highs and lows and the hormonal shifts, there is power in that. But we were taught to be ashamed of it and not even seek to understand it or explore it for our own edification, let alone to help the next generation."
~ Michelle Obama

Your forties came, and there is no sign of perimenopause anywhere. Then came your fifties, and that pesky monthly visitor never misses a beat. Your period is exactly the same as it has been for the past few decades. What gives? You could be one of the women in the world who are experiencing late menopause.

Menopause usually occurs between the ages of forty-five and fifty-five. The average age is about fifty-one. Late-onset menopause occurs after the age of fifty-five. There is no need to worry if all of your friends are talking about their personal summers and night sweats while you are still having to tote feminine products everywhere you go. According to Alloy Staff (2022), there are benefits to late-onset menopause.

Benefits

<u>Reduced risk of osteoporosis</u> – Estrogen helps to keep your bones strong. If your body continues to produce estrogen longer, it stands to reason that your bones will be stronger and healthier. This means that they are less likely to break or fracture, which helps you maintain a healthy, active lifestyle.

<u>Reduced risk of heart disease and stroke</u> – Estrogen not only helps bones, but it also helps protect the heart muscle and the circulatory system. When your body continues to produce estrogen later in your life, your heart and circulatory system are protected much longer. According to Alloy Staff (2022), women who have late-onset menopause are two percent less likely to suffer from heart disease or to have a stroke due to plaque-clogged arteries.

<u>Increased life span</u> – Interestingly enough, you could add a couple of years to your life if you are experiencing late menopause. There have been several studies that indicate that if you have late onset menopause, then you have a longer life span than other women. You will live, on average, two years longer than women who start menopause before they are forty.

· · ·

Risks

Although there are some awesome benefits to late menopause, it doesn't come without risks. Faris (2017) states that one of the risks of late-onset menopause is an increased danger of certain cancers, such as breast, ovarian, and uterine. The heightened risk is because your body is producing estrogen longer. Therefore, you must have regular pelvic exams, pap smears, and mammograms

Causes

Several risk factors can delay the onset of menopause (Jones, 2022).

<u>Genetics</u> -- According to Jones (2022), genetics is most influential on when you will experience menopause – approximately fifty percent of the time.

<u>Obesity</u> – If you are overweight or considered to be obese then you are fifty percent more likely to experience late menopause than other women. This is because estrogen is produced and stored in the fat tissues, which puts off the time when estrogen levels decrease.

<u>Menstrual cycle</u> – If you started your period late or it was irregular, you may experience late menopause. If your body had naturally higher levels of estrogen, then menopause may be delayed.

<u>Pregnancies</u> – The number of pregnancies you've had and the timing of those pregnancies can affect when you experience menopause. This includes whether you've had at least one baby, had multiple pregnancies, had one baby later in life, or your first pregnancy was later in life.

<u>Diet</u> – Your diet is one of the considerations that can affect menopause. If you eat a lot of fruit, vegetables, and proteins, menopause might be delayed. If you eat meat, then menopause might come later than vegetarians' menopause. Eating a lot of fish and fresh legumes may also cause a delay in the onset of menopause by more than three years. Taking in higher amounts of Vitamin B6 or zinc may also cause a slight delay in the onset of menopause. On the flip side, diets that are full of carbohydrates, like pasta and rice, may experience early-onset menopause.

<u>Alcohol</u> – There is a correlation between regular alcohol consumption and when you experience menopause.

<u>Birth control</u> – Studies indicate that if you have taken birth control, you might experience late-onset menopause.

<u>Thyroid</u> – According to Faris (2017), some thyroid disorders can also delay menopause.

Symptoms

The symptoms for late menopause are the same as they are for perimenopause and menopause. You may experience hot flashes, night sweats, trouble sleeping, vaginal dryness, and all of the other symptoms. Like perimenopause and menopause, not everyone experiences these the same. They might come in slowly and subtly so you don't notice them. On the other hand, they might be so intense that they interrupt the quality of your life. If the latter is the case, you will want to have a candid conversation with your doctor to determine what solutions are available.

. . .

Hormone Replacement Therapy

Hormone replacement therapy (HRT) is an option if you are experiencing late menopause and your symptoms interfere with your quality of life. It can help alleviate the symptoms and protect against osteoporosis, heart disease, and the risk of stroke. We will discuss the benefits and risks of HRT in the next chapter. Because there are some risks, you should talk to your doctor about whether HRT is right for you.

Pregnancy

According to Faris (2017), it is imperative to remember that you can still get pregnant if you are experiencing late menopause. Pregnancies are possible until you have gone a full twelve months without any period. Therefore, unless you don't mind a surprise, you should continue taking birth control or using contraceptives.

When to Consult Your Doctor

Just as it is with perimenopause or regular menopause, there may be a time when you should talk to your doctor. A lot of women can handle the symptoms of menopause. However, for other women, they can be so severe that it interferes with their quality of life. After all, it is hard to get up, take care of your family, go to work, and do your day-to-day chores when you cannot sleep, your migraines are killing you, and you look like you just stepped out of a sauna every ten minutes. Your doctor can help suggest lifestyle changes or medications that can mitigate the severity of these symptoms so that your life can return to some semblance of normalcy.

Conclusion

My father used to tell me all the time that knowledge is power. The adage is true. My mother told me about when she first experienced her period. She started when she was in her sixth-grade class. In her time, no one talked about such things, so she was terrified when it happened and had no idea what to do. Luckily, times have changed, and she knew what to expect when she hit menopause.

Knowing and understanding the changes that you are experiencing can help alleviate any fear that you might be experiencing and help you find the tools to deal with the experiences. Knowledge about the symptoms that accompany this transition gives you the power to control them and how you feel as you go through another transition in your life. I hope this book, so far, is giving you the knowledge to feel more in control of what is happening in your body.

One of the most important topics of conversation surrounding menopause, regardless of what stage you are in, is hormone replacement therapy. In the next chapter, we will discuss what hormone replacement therapy is, the risks, the benefits, and whether it is right for you.

Stand up and stretch. Grab a drink and then settle back in as you journey through the world of estrogen, progesterone, and bioidentical hormones.

Chapter 4

Hormone Replacement Therapy

"One thing I love about aging - and I do love aging - I've got a wisdom that no young person can buy. You earn it."
~Suzanne Somers

You've had enough. The hot flashes are so bad that sweat is soaking through your clothes. You want to have those special moments with your partner, but your libido has decreased to nothingness, and the vaginal dryness makes it uncomfortable or even painful. Your motivation has run out of gas. When symptoms of perimenopause and menopause become too much and interfere with your quality of life, it is time to talk to your doctor. Hormone replacement therapy is an option that your doctor may discuss with you either during perimenopause or menopause.

As you know, during perimenopause, your estrogen levels can rise and fall. Then, during menopause, they continue to fall as your ovaries are no longer producing the hormone. This can cause you to experience some unpleasant symptoms. Hormone replacement therapy (HRT) is an option that can help. It is a medication that contains female hormones. Your doctor might prescribe medication that only contains estrogen or they might decide to prescribe medication that has both estrogen and progesterone therapy (WebMD, 2023).

Estrogen hormone replacement therapy would be prescribed if you have gone through perimenopause or menopause and have had a hysterectomy -- whether you've only had your uterus removed or your ovaries have been removed as well. If you still have your uterus, your doctor will likely prescribe a therapy containing estrogen and progesterone. This is because when you only take estrogen and you still have your uterus, then the hormone might cause the lining on your uterus to grow, which, in turn, can lead to endometrial cancer. Progesterone helps to prevent the thickening of the uterine lining (Mayo Clinic, 2023; Medline Plus, 2023).

Estrogen therapy

Estrogen hormone replacement therapy is when the doctor prescribes medication that only has the one hormone. This hormone plays an important role helping to regulate your body. According to the Cleveland Clinic (2023), estrogen helps to:

1. Thicken the lining in your uterus
2. Influence the use of calcium in your body
3. Maintain healthy cholesterol levels
4. Make sure your vagina stays healthy
5. Works to prevent osteoporosis

<u>Hormone therapy types</u>

There are two ways estrogen-only hormone replacement therapy is administered. The first is systematic hormone therapy. The estrogen may come as a pill, patch, gel, ring, cream, or a spray foam. This method usually has higher levels of estrogen and is absorbed throughout your body. This method can be used to treat the most common side effects that you experience due to menopause (Mayo Clinic, 2023).

The second way that estrogen is administered is vaginally in low doses. These might come in a vaginal tablet, cream, or ring. This minimizes the amount of estrogen that is absorbed in the body. This type of therapy is used mainly to treat vaginal issues and prevent potential urinary tract infections (Mayo Clinic, 2023).

<u>Benefits</u>

There are a lot of benefits of estrogen therapy (WebMD, 2023). It can help decrease hot flashes, night sweats, help you sleep better, decrease vaginal discomfort, decrease pain during sex, help prevent osteoporosis, and decrease chances of dementia and heart disease.

<u>Side effects</u>

Just like any other type of medical treatment or therapies, there are side effects that you could experience when you are taking just estrogen therapy. You should monitor for the following issues and contact your doctor if you experience any of them (WebMD, 2023).

· Bloating

· Breast pain or tenderness

· Mood changes

· Nausea

· Vaginal bleeding or discharge

Progesterone therapy

Progesterone is the other female hormone that is created in your ovaries, and will decrease during menopause. Many times, if you are going through menopause but you still have your uterus, you will be treated with both estrogen and progesterone. However, sometimes progesterone is prescribed by itself. This might happen if the estrogen levels are steady. It might also be prescribed by itself because it has many benefits on its own (Belcher, 2023).

<u>How progesterone is administered</u>

You would normally take progesterone in the form of a tablet around bedtime. You must take the medication at the same time every day so you don't forget. According to Medline Plus (2023), you will likely take the hormone on a rotating schedule. You would take them for ten to twelve days and then take a break from the treatment for sixteen to eighteen days. Your doctor will let you know exactly how and when to take the medication. It is important that you take the medication exactly as the instructions tell you.

Don't take it any more or less than is prescribed. If you start to have odd symptoms or you start to feel unwell after you have taken it, call your doctor.

<u>Benefits</u>

According to Dr. Leigh Ann Scott (Leighannscottmd.com, 2023), progesterone is thought by some people to be a miracle hormone because it helps to calm both the mind and the body. When your progesterone levels are low, you might experience mood swings, depression, or increased anxiety. It also helps to stimulate your brain processes and aids in the proper functioning of your nervous system. There are many benefits to taking this hormone.

1. Prepares uterus for the fertilized egg to be implanted

2. Regulate blood pressure

3. Improves your mood

4. Improves your sleep

5. Improves memory

6. Decreases anxiety

7. Protects you from the overgrowth of certain types of cells, preventing certain cancers such as breast and uterine cancer

8. Decreases risk of fibrocystic disease and helps prevents ovarian cysts.

9. Increases your ability to handle stress

10. Helps to prevent the lining of the uterus from thickening too much, thereby preventing endometriosis

11. Promotes bone growth

12. Reduces weight gain

13. Decreases hot flashes

14. Reduces joint pain and inflammation of joints.

15. Improves your sex drive.

16. Helps promote your metabolism

17. Helps to prevent the plaque from growing on your arterial walls.

18. Slows the aging process

19. Helps the thyroid to function correctly

20. Helps to prevent diabetes

<u>Side Effects</u>

Medline Plus (2023) lists several side effects that might be caused by the progesterone. If they become severe or if they persist, then you need to call your doctor as soon as possible. These side effects include:

· Fatigue

· Runny nose

· Cough

· Sneezing

· Vaginal discharge

· Difficulty with urination

· Headaches

· Nausea

· Vomiting

· Diarrhea

· Constipation

· Irritability

· Tender breasts or breast pain

· Excessive worrying

· Mood swings

· Muscle, joint, or bone pain

You might experience some serious side effects when you are taking progesterone. If any of these occur, you should call your doctor immediately.

· Lumps on your breasts

· Migraines

· Hoarseness

· Problems breathing or swallowing

· Swelling of your face, throat, tongue, eyes, hands, feet, ankles, lips, or lower legs

· Rash

· Itching

· Hives

· Stomach pain or swelling of the stomach

· Seizures

· Depression

· Seeing double

· Vaginal bleeding that is unexpected

· Uncontrollable shaking hands

· Bulging eyes

· Loss of vision or blurred vision

· Coughing up blood

· Swelling legs or pain in your legs

· Sharp chest pain

· Fast heart rate

· Shortness of breath

· Incoordination or loss of balance

· Weakness and/ or numbness in the upper legs and arms

· Slow or difficult speech

· Dizziness or faintness that becomes severe

According to Medline Plus (2023), tumors developed in animals that took the progesterone, although scientists are not sure whether the hormone will cause tumors to grow in humans.

Another risk of taking progesterone is that it is known to cause blood clots. This is very dangerous because it can cause the blood supply to be cut off to your brain, heart, lungs, and other organs.

Benefits of Combined HRT

There have been several studies regarding the benefits and dangers of partaking in hormone replacement therapy. Some of the benefits are: (National Cancer Institute, 2023).

<u>Hip and vertebrae fractures</u> – The studies showed that women who took either estrogen HRT or estrogen and progesterone HRT had a decreased risk of suffering from either a hip or vertebrae fracture. This benefit no longer existed if the women stopped taking the HRT.

<u>Breast cancer</u> – Women who took estrogen alone showed a decreased risk of breast cancer.

The Mayo Clinic (2023) states that there are other benefits to HRT.

<u>Moderate to severe hot flashes</u> – Systemic estrogen therapy is the best way to treat hot flashes and night sweats.

<u>Ease vaginal discomfort</u> – This includes dryness, itchiness, burning, and pain during intercourse.

<u>Treat symptoms of early menopause</u> – Estrogen might be recommended by your doctor if you had a full hysterectomy wherein you had your ovaries removed as well as your uterus, because your body hasn't received all of the estrogen other women have had and that is necessary for good health. You might also be given estrogen if your ovaries were not functioning properly and weren't creating enough estrogen for you. The estrogen treatments can help prevent dementia, mood changes, stroke, heart disease, and other health issues.

Negative Effects of Combined HRT

The studies that were conducted on women who were taking HRT versus those who were taking placebos also showed that there were negative side effects of the HRT (National Cancer Institute, 2023).

<u>Vaginal bleeding</u> – According to National Cancer Institute (2023), some women who were taking HRT that included both estrogen and progesterone had vaginal bleeding that needed an endometrial biopsy.

<u>Incontinence</u> – The studies also showed that women who took HRT that had both hormones had an increased risk of incontinence.

<u>Dementia</u> – Women who took HRT and were sixty-five years or older were at a higher risk of developing dementia.

Stroke, blood clots, and heart attack – Women who took only estrogen or estrogen and progesterone showed an increase risk of stroke, blood clots, and heart attacks. However, these risks returned to normal once the women stopped taking the HRT.

Breast Cancer – Women who were going through HRT and took both estrogen and progesterone had an increased risk of breast cancer. In addition, it is likely that the cancer spread to the lymph nodes by the time it was diagnosed. The risk sharply decreases once the HRT is stopped. To make matters worse, mammograms are not as effective at detecting cancer in women who are going through HRT, whether it is just estrogen or both hormones.

Lung cancer – The risk of developing lung cancer is no different between the women who were taking both estrogen and progesterone compared to those who were taking the placebo. However, women undergoing HRT were more likely to die from the disease.

Colorectal cancer – This one is a mixed bag. National Cancer Institute (2023) stated that women who took the combined therapy had a lower risk of colorectal cancer. However, the tumors, when they appeared, were more advanced than the tumors suffered by the placebo group. The increased risk returned to normal once the women stopped taking the combined HRT. Women who were taking just the estrogen had the same risk and stage of cancer as those who took the placebo.

It is important to remember that there are different

factors that will help determine your risk of cancer, heart disease, strokes, blood clots, etc (Mayo Clinic, 2023). These include:

· Age – You will be at a higher risk if you start the hormone therapy when you are sixty years old or older, or if you start taking it more than ten years after menopause begins. However, by taking the therapy before age sixty or before you hit that ten year benchmark then the benefits seem to outweigh the risks.

· Type of therapy – the risks depend on whether you are taking estrogen alone or if you are taking the combined therapy of estrogen and progesterone. In addition, it also depends on how the estrogen is administered and how much is being given.

· Health history – Your health history and that of your family's has an important impact on whether you are at greater risk for some conditions.

Reducing the Risks

You've talked to your doctor about what is going on with your body and you both agree that hormone replacement therapy would be the best course for you. The good news is that although there are certain risks of hormone replacement therapy, there are ways to mitigate the risks (Mayo Clinic, 2023).

1. You and your doctor should determine the best product and the best way to deliver that product. For example, if you really aren't suffering too much from hot flashes but the vaginal discomforts are making life a little hard to

enjoy, then estrogen might be the best solution, and the best way to administer it might be through a vaginal cream.

2. Take the minimal amount of medication needed for the least amount of time. You might have to take larger amounts of the hormones for longer time periods if you are younger than forty-five, and the purpose of taking it is to prevent negative long-term health effects. Longer treatments might also be recommended if your symptoms of menopause are decreasing your quality of life.

3. Regular follow-up care – You should see your doctor on a regular basis to ensure that the benefits are still outweighing the risks. You will also want to get regular preventive care, such as pelvic examinations and mammograms.

4. Choose a healthy lifestyle – It is important that you exercise regularly and that you eat right. Don't smoke, and limit the amount of alcohol that you drink. Ensure that you are managing your stress well. You should also ensure that you are monitoring your health conditions, such as high blood pressure.

When HRT Is NOT Right for You

Although there are several reasons why you might want to consider HRT, National Health Services (2023) lists several conditions that make HRT unsuitable.

1. Liver disease or liver tumors
2. You are pregnant
3. Untreated high blood pressure
4. History of blood clots

5. History of uterine cancer, breast cancer, or ovarian cancer

6. History of endometrial cancer

7. History of active deep vein thrombosis or a pulmonary embolism

8. Unexplained vaginal bleeding

9. If you smoke, HRT could increase your risk for blood clots or strokes

Difference Between Natural Hormones and Hormones Used in HRT

The difference between the natural hormones and the hormones used in HRT is that the hormones used in HRT are made from different plants and animals, or they could be created synthetically in a laboratory. National Cancer Institute (2023) stated that the hormones produced in the lab or from plants and animals are similar to the hormones that you produce naturally, but are not exactly the same.

Bioidentical hormones

The term bioidentical refers to the fact that these hormones are chemically the same as the hormones produced by your body. A lot of these are very similar to the ones that are produced in laboratories and prescribed to you by your doctor, although they still must be processed commercially before they are ready to be used. Many of the bioidentical hormones are approved by the Food and Drug Administration (Burnett, 2023).

Some of the bioidentical hormones used in hormone replacement therapy are not approved by the FDA. These hormones are widely sold on the internet. You do not need a prescription to purchase these hormones. The purveyors of these hormones will often say that they are safer and more effective than those approved by the FDA, although those claims have not been proven.

One difference between those that are not approved by the FDA is that they come in different doses and forms that are not consistent with those that are approved by the FDA. According to Burnett (2023), the ones that are approved by the FDA have to go through a compounding pharmacy. However, the ones sold on the internet without a prescription are not always held up to the same high-quality standards.

Another difference is that some of the bioidentical hormones that are not FDA approved are custom-made for you. The amount needed is based on a saliva test. Unfortunately, your saliva does not accurately depict the level of hormones in your blood (Burnett, 2023).

Bioidentical hormones that you can get over the counter are not necessarily pure. While those that are FDA approved are guaranteed to have been created safely, there is no such guarantee with those that have not been approved. In essence, you have only the maker's word that these products are pure and safe. According to the Cleveland Clinic (2023), over-the-counter hormones might contain additional hormones than just what is advertised.

You should talk to your doctor if you are thinking about going this route because of the risks entailed. There are more than a million women who have used these products safely and with great satisfaction. However, before jumping into the deep end with both feet, you need to analyze the risks and benefits and determine whether they are the right solution for you. Always err on the side of caution when starting any new medication and discuss it with your physician.

Conclusion

I know that I just threw a lot of heavy information at you, but I feel that it is so important that you have all the facts that you need when you talk to your doctor about hormone replacement therapy. The first step is to determine what symptoms you are dealing with and whether they affect your quality of life.

If you decide that hormone replacement therapy might be the way to go, you should weigh the benefits of taking only estrogen, only progesterone, or both. It is very important that you understand the benefits of each, the risks of each, and whether the benefits outweigh the risks.

Another important thing to consider centers on bioidentical hormones. They are chemically the same as those produced naturally by your body. However, there is a difference between those that the FDA approves and those that are not.

This is your life and health, and it is important that you aren't risking it on a roll of the dice. Carefully consider all of your options. As a matter of fact, why don't you grab that pen and paper and make a pro and con list? On one side, write why you think hormone replacement therapy might be right for you. On the other side, write why you think you might forgo HRT. Then, see if the pros outweigh the cons.

When you are ready, sit down and buckle your seat belt as we continue our journey to the next chapter to talk about ways to alleviate the symptoms of menopause by focusing on lifestyle changes.

Chapter 5

Alternatives Ways to Mitigate Symptoms, Lifestyle Changes, Support Groups, and More

"And the beauty of a woman, with passing years only grows!"
~ Audrey Hepburn

As you sweat through the next ten minutes, feeling like you have become one with the sun, you think that there has to be some kind of solution that can help you get through those endless sleepless nights and other symptoms that have taken over your life – a solution that doesn't involve the standard medical treatments.

Alternative Treatment

There are quite a few alternative treatments you can consider if you decide that hormone replacement therapy or the other prescribed drugs aren't quite what you want right now. However, there are times when your symptoms can make your life almost unbearable. Make sure that you talk to your doctor before using alternative treatments.

<u>Phytoestrogens</u>

Phytoestrogens are hormones that occur naturally in some plants. According to the Mayo Clinic (2023), two types of phytoestrogens can be found in plants – isoflavones and lignans. The estrogen you get from eating these plants mimics the estrogen your body produces naturally.

According to White and Cherney (2021), one benefit of eating phytoestrogen-rich foods, such as soy, is that they can help decrease the frequency and severity of hot flashes. Studies have also indicated that consuming phytoestrogens can help decrease the risks of losing bone density, which in turn, helps decrease the chances of osteoporosis.

Phytoestrogens can also help with menstrual issues when you are in the perimenopausal stage. Because estrogen levels fluctuate, phytoestrogens can help level out the hormone levels and help mitigate menstruation irregularities during this time (White and Cherney 2021).

My favorite part of getting out of puberty was that I had less acne. Then, when I started going through peri-menopause, those nasty pimples showed back up. This is because estrogen levels are decreasing, and androgens – male hormones – are increasing. Therefore, one solution to the problem is to eat foods that are rich in phytoestrogens (White and Cherney, 2021).

White and Cherney (2021) state that one study found

that consuming soy helped decrease incidences of breast cancer and death associated with it. Research has also indicated that phytoestrogens positively impact the diagnosis and prognosis of endometrial and colorectal cancer.

Studies have indicated that phytoestrogens can positively affect your health in other areas. For example, one study showed that consuming phytoestrogens decreases high blood pressure as well as type 2 diabetes. Another study showed that women who consumed phytoestrogens had a decreased risk of heart disease and dementia (White and Cherney, 2021).

Risks

According to White and Cherney (2021), you need to talk to your doctor if you decide to eat phytoestrogen, as there can be some risks. Although the risks haven't been proven in clinical studies, there has been some conjecture that taking phytoestrogens – whether you eat them or take a supplement – can cause health issues, such as obesity, heart disease, cancer, and reproductive disorders.

Food and herbs rich in phytoestrogens

There are many foods and herbs that are rich in phytoestrogens, and of course, some contain higher amounts than others. You can also take supplements that can help increase your estrogen levels. The supplements normally have higher amounts of the hormones than plants, so use them with care. The following plants are known to have phytoestrogens:

- Soy
- Licorice root
- Angelica
- Carrots
- Broccoli
- Black cohosh
- Dong quai
- Coffee
- Chaste tree berry
- Angelia
- Evening primrose
- Oranges
- Red clover
- Tea
- Legumes
- Dark chocolate
- Vitamin D
- Garlic oil supplements
- Flax seeds
- Omega-3 fatty acids
- Tofu
- Sesame seeds
- Beans
- Linseeds
- Tempeh

Caution

There are no known side effects of consuming plants that contain phytoestrogens. If you like broccoli and carrots, then eat your heart out. However, if you are thinking about taking phytoestrogens as a supplement, you need to talk to your doctor and do your research on the product. These supplements are not regulated by the FDA. This means the purity level, quality, and dosage are not guaranteed. You will want to look at the companies that sell the supplements to determine which ones have the best reputation for high-quality products before you make the plunge. White and Cherney (2021) recommend that you try getting the phytoestrogen boosts naturally from the food before you think about taking the supplements.

Black cohosh

I wanted to discuss this particular supplement individually because it does seem to be a very popular alternative treatment for menopausal symptoms. It is a member of the buttercup family and has been used by Native Americans for centuries. Menopausal women use it to help reduce the frequency and severity of hot flashes and other symptoms (NIH, 2020).

There have been many studies on the effects of black cohosh on menopausal symptoms, and there seem to be mixed results. Part of the issue is a difference in the dosage of the supplement, as well as the formula, plant species, and other such issues. In some clinical trials, women have been able to take the supplement for a full year and haven't had any harmful side effects. However, there have been reports of liver damage, sometimes severe, with some commercial black cohosh products. The National Institute of Health (NIH) stated that these instances were rare and it was unclear whether the individuals suffered liver problems because of the supplement or because they already had liver problems. It is very important that you check with a doctor before taking this supplement if you do have liver problems.

In addition to liver problems, some women suffered other side effects when taking the supplement. These side effects include nausea, cramps, rashes, headaches, weight gain, vaginal spotting or bleeding, and a feeling of heaviness. You should talk to your doctor if you have any of these symptoms (NIH, 2020).

If you decide that you do want to try this supplement, then you need to make sure that you research the company that sells it. According to NIH (2020), research found that some commercially sold products had the wrong herb in them – it wasn't black cohosh at all. Another issue was that some of the products included additional herbs that were not listed on the label.

As with any supplement that you take, whether it is for the relief of menopausal symptoms or other issues, make sure that you talk to your doctor before you start them.

Bioidentical hormones

We talked about these in the last chapter, but as a

reminder, bioidentical hormones are plant-based supplements that can provide estrogen and progesterone. The plants go through a chemical process to ensure that the hormones are the same as those produced by your body. There are some bioidentical hormones that have been tested and have been approved by the FDA (Mayo Clinic, 2023).

The concern comes when the hormones are compounded or prepared by a pharmacist in accordance with a doctor's prescriptions. Because these supplements aren't monitored by the FDA, the dosage and quality of the products cannot be guaranteed. The Mayo Clinic (2023) states that there is no evidence that bioidentical hormones work any better than hormone replacement therapy. There is also no evidence to suggest that these supplements are any less risky than HRT.

Lifestyle Changes

As we discussed, hormone replacement therapy is one treatment option for your perimenopausal and menopausal symptoms. Other types of medications, such as SSRIs, are also an option. However, alternative solutions can help mitigate the severity of your symptoms. Some are easy lifestyle changes, while others might be a little more challenging but not impossible. Are you ready to take back control of your life?

Diet to treat symptoms

This was an extremely hard one for me. I enjoy my cherry cheesecake pastries and my white bread. I love spicy food, and everyone enjoys me more when I've had caffeine in the morning. However, making a few changes in your diet can significantly affect the severity and frequency of your symptoms.

<u>Dairy</u>

Estrogen is an important hormone for bone health. When your body produces normal levels of estrogen, the hormone tells your bones not to break down. However, once your estrogen levels decrease, then so does your bone density. This can lead to painful, and sometimes serious, breaks and fractures. It can also lead to osteoporosis (2018).

However, consuming dairy products, such as milk, yogurt, and cheese all contain important vitamins and minerals that are essential for bone health, such as calcium, potassium, phosphorus, magnesium, vitamin D, and vitamin K. Groves (2018) stated that one study of almost seven hundred and fifty women showed that postmenopausal women who had substantially higher bone density consumed more dairy products and proteins than their counterparts who ate less.

Dairy products aren't just good for helping to increase bone density. Studies have indicated that consuming dairy products can also help improve sleep. According to Groves (2018), one study indicated that food with high amounts of the amino acid glycine helped menopausal women sleep more deeply. This particular amino acid is found in milk and cheese, as well as other dairy products (Groves, 2018).

The best part is that ice cream does qualify for dairy

products. There are some ice cream brands out there that are low in sugar and still taste delicious.

<u>Healthy fat</u>

Do you like fish? If so, this will be exciting news for you. A study of more than four hundred and eighty women indicated that the omega-3 fatty acids helped decrease the frequency women suffered from hot flashes. The fatty acids also helped decrease the severity of night sweats. If you are like me and fish isn't one of your favorites, then you can take supplements and get the same benefits (Groves, 2018). Salmon, mackerel, and anchovies are just a few of the fish that have high amounts of this healthy fat.

<u>Whole grains</u>

Whole grains are very important. As your estrogen levels decrease, your risk for heart disease, stroke, cancer, and diabetes increases. Eating whole grains, such as brown rice, whole-wheat bread, barley, rye, and quinoa can help decrease your risks of these potentially fatal diseases. That is because they are rich in fiber, vitamin B, niacin, thiamine, riboflavin, and pantothenic acid (Groves, 2018).

Groves (2018) cited one study of more than eleven hundred postmenopausal women who ate almost five grams of whole-grain fiber per their two thousand calorie diet and reduced their risks of dying early by seventeen percent, compared to women who only consumed a little more than a gram of whole-grain fiber with the same diet.

In addition, another study showed that eating a daily serving of at least three servings of whole grains had a twenty to thirty percent decrease in the risk of diabetes and heart disease (Groves, 2018).

<u>Protein</u>

Unfortunately, a decline in estrogen is also responsible for a decrease in muscle mass. The good news is that food rich in protein can help. In addition, high-protein diets also help with bone strength. According to the recommended daily allowance, ten to thirty-five percent of your daily calorie intake should be protein. Women who are going through menopause or are post-menopausal should eat about half a gram of protein per one pound of their body weight, which equals out to be around twenty-five grams of protein per meal (Groves, 2018).

One large study showed that women who were over fifty and who ate the recommended amount of dairy proteins had an eight percent decreased risk of hip fractures. Those who ate the recommended amount of plant-based proteins showed a twelve percent reduced risk (Groves, 2018).

Foods that are high in proteins include eggs, dairy products, meat, fish, and legumes. Peanut butter is a terrific source of protein if you happen to like peanut butter spread on whole-wheat bread as a snack. You can also get proteins in powder form. I like to start my mornings off with a protein shake.

<u>Calcium and vitamin D</u>

Because there is a direct link between decreased estrogen levels and lower bone density, osteoporosis is a significant concern. However, consuming foods that are high in calcium can help mitigate bone loss and decrease your risk for fractures and breaks. Not only are dairy products good for calcium, but other foods such as kale, spinach, collard greens, sardines, tofu, beans, and other foods are high in calcium, naturally. You can also consume food products that are fortified with calcium, such as juices and cereal products (Brown, 2022).

Vitamin D is also necessary to fortify your bone density as it helps your body to absorb calcium. A great source of vitamin D is sunlight because your skin produces the vitamin when you are in the sun. Foods rich in this vitamin include oily fish, eggs, and cod liver oil, as well as foods that are fortified with the vitamin. You can also take vitamin D as a supplement (Brown, 2022).

<u>Fruits and vegetables</u>

Lucky for me, I love a lot of different kinds of fruits and vegetables. Not only are some fruits and vegetables rich in phytoestrogen, but they also have other minerals and vitamins that are helpful in alleviating some of the symptoms associated with menopause. For example, thy can help you to maintain a healthy weight, which can be an issue for menopausal and postmenopausal women. Maintaining a healthy weight can decrease instances of high blood pressure, heart disease, and diabetes. Fruits and vegetables also help decrease your risk of heart disease and bone loss (Brown, 2022).

<u>Foods to avoid</u>

I know – everyone is trying to take away your favorite

foods for one reason or another. It can be so hard to avoid them. You see other people eating these types of foods. Your taste buds are ready to enjoy just a few bites of pastry or spicy Mexican food. But then you sadly tell yourself to stop drooling over what you can't have. This is all because of menopause. Some types of food can make the symptoms of menopause worse. Therefore, if you avoid the foods, your symptoms might decrease in severity.

Sugars and processed carbs

These foods can contribute to high blood sugar, insulin resistance, and metabolic syndrome, which has been related to hot flashes. These foods have been shown to rapidly raise your blood sugar levels. The more processed the food is, the faster your blood sugar will increase. If you limit these foods, such as white bread and crackers, and other baked goodies and processed foods, your hot flashes may come less often and not be as severe. According to Groves (2018) sugar intake should be less than ten percent of your daily calories.

Alcohol and caffeine

There is nothing more relaxing than a glass of sweet wine after dinner, and nothing gets me going in the morning better than a Suisse mocha – or three. However, both alcohol and caffeine have been linked to hot flashes. Therefore, limiting your intake of these substances may help decrease the severity of your personal summers (Groves, 2018).

In addition, both of these have been shown to disrupt sleep. Therefore, if you are struggling to sleep, you might consider not indulging in these drinks for a couple of hours before bedtime.

Spicy food

This breaks my heart because I love spicy food. Some studies have indicated a link between spicy food and hot flashes. Another study showed a link between spicy food and anxiety levels (Groves, 2018).

Sodium-rich food

Research has indicated that high salt intake may lower your bone density. One study that included almost ten thousand postmenopausal women indicated that if you consume more than two grams of salt each day, you are likely to be twenty-eight percent more likely to have lower bone density. In addition, decreasing your salt intake can also decrease your risk of high blood pressure (Groves, 2018).

According to Groves (2018), one study showed that decreasing salt intake may help you be in a better mood.

<u>Keep a food and symptom diary</u>

Because certain foods might trigger hot flashes, insomnia, or one of the other symptoms of menopause Brown (2022) suggests that you keep a food and symptom diary. No two women go through the process exactly the same, which means the foods that trigger your best friend's symptoms aren't necessarily going to trigger yours. You might be able to eat spicy foods and not experience hot flashes at all. On the other hand, if she so much as looks at a jalapeño pepper, she turns into a burning furnace. By keeping a journal, you can see how your activities either cause some of the symptoms to show up or help alleviate them.

Maintain a healthy weight

This topic goes under lifestyle changes because menopause can cause us to gain weight. Before I hit menopause, I could pretty much eat anything and still maintain my girlish figure. As soon as menopause hit, I gained almost thirty pounds. It seemed as though this weight appeared overnight. It was clear that my lifestyle before perimenopause and menopause wouldn't work for me now.

Spritzler (2021) states several factors that can lead to weight gain due to menopause. One is that you are not sleeping as well as you should, and a lack of sleep leads to weight gain. Women tend to suffer from increased insulin resistance as they age, which in turn, contributes to weight gain. You are also more subject to weight gain when your hormones fluctuate. A loss of muscle mass increases the risk of weight gain. If that isn't enough, Spritzler (2021) says that the fat stored in your hips and thighs shifts to your abdomen.

The problem is that when you gain weight, especially around your waist, there is an increased risk of heart disease and diabetes. Body weight also has an impact on your symptoms associated with menopause. Brown (2022) reports that a study of more than seventeen thousand postmenopausal women found that the women who lost at least ten pounds, or ten percent of their body weight over the course of a year experienced fewer instances of hot flashes and night sweats.

<u>Calories</u>

Calories is kind of a frightening word because the second that we hear it, we automatically start ticking off everything that we've eaten for the day and how many calories our food contained. We feel guilty if we ate too much. Unfortunately, to lose weight, we need to decrease the amount of calories that we take in.

Spritzler (2021) states that when you reach menopause, you will burn fewer calories when you are at rest than you did when you were premenopausal. To combat this, you might be tempted to try a very low-calorie diet to lose weight. However, severely cutting the number of calories you consume can backfire. Research has indicated that restricting your diet so that you consume low-calorie levels can make you lose muscle mass and decrease your metabolism. This can make it even harder to keep the weight off. Quickly losing weight due to a severe decline in calories can also lead to a significant decline in bone density, increasing your risk for osteoporosis.

Instead of going on a low-calorie diet to try to lose weight quickly, Spritzler (2021) suggests a low-carbohydrate diet. She cites one study that indicates that postmenopausal women on a low-carb diet lost approximately twenty-two pounds, almost twenty-eight percent of their body fat, and three and a half inches of fat from their waist over six months.

The Mediterranean diet not only helps reduce the risk of heart disease and increases your overall health, but it can also help you lose weight. A vegetarian diet can help you lose weight and may also help decrease the frequency and severity of hot flashes. Vegetarian diets that include dairy products and eggs have been proven to work well with post-menopausal women (Spritzler, 2021).

<u>Diet tips</u>

Spritzler (2021) has several diet tips to help you lose weight.

Protein

A diet that includes protein-rich foods can help you lose weight. Protein has been shown to help you feel fuller and more satisfied. It also decreases the loss of muscle mass and increases your metabolism.

Dairy

According to Spritzler (2021), consuming dairy products while you are trying to lose weight can help you maintain your muscle mass while, at the same time, helping you lose fat.

Soluble fiber

It is a good idea to eat foods rich in soluble fiber. This includes food such as Brussels sprouts, avocados, and broccoli. These foods can help increase insulin sensitivity and reduce your appetite.

Green tea

Drinking green tea contains caffeine and epigallocatechin gallate that helps you burn fat.

Mindful eating

Mindful eating is when you use all of your senses to enjoy the foods that you eat. Spritzler (2021) states that this can help improve your relationship with food and reduce your stress. The result is that you eat less.

<u>Exercises</u>

Exercising, of course, is a great way to help you lose that belly fat and to keep your weight in check. According to Spritzler (2021), there are two types of exercises that are most helpful. One is resistance training with either bands or weights. This type of exercise can help you preserve and even increase your muscle mass. Research indicates that the more repetitions you do, the more abdominal fat you will lose. Aerobic exercises, or cardio exercises, are also great for helping to reduce abdominal fat, maintain muscle mass, and even increase your muscle mass. For best results, you should combine the two types of exercises.

When Morpheus Eludes You

When I was younger, I loved to stay up until two or three o'clock in the morning. I wasn't even a party girl. I liked watching television, reading books, and even working on crafts. Now, though, eleven rolls around, and all I want is my bed. I'm tired. My eyes are heavy. I can't focus on my project.

I get ready for bed – the usual – I brush my teeth, comb my hair, change into my jammies, and crawl in between my sheets. And then, my eyes pop wide open. I can't sleep. Or, I'm able to go to sleep for a couple of hours, and then I wake up around two or three in the morning and I can't go back to sleep. Then, there are the nights I can sleep, but it isn't restful. It seems that I have a stalker, and his name is insomnia.

It is one of the more common symptoms associated with menopause. Sometimes it is because you have night sweats, and sometimes it is just because you can't sleep. A lack of sleep can wreak havoc in your life. You are unable to focus on tasks and you can't concentrate. It affects your memory, like you suddenly can't remember why you walked into the kitchen. I've had a hard time staying awake during the day. I'll be working at my desk, and all of a sudden, I have an overwhelming need for a nap.

In addition to all the other problems associated with insomnia, there is a correlation between a lack of sleep and weight gain (Spritzler, 2021). People who don't get enough sleep tend to have higher levels of ghrelin, a hunger hormone. They also have lower levels of leptin, which tells you when you are full.

Causes

<u>Hormones</u>

According to Dr. Heather Currie (2021), there are several factors that may be contributing to your inability to sleep. One is your hormones, which cause hot flashes and night sweats. No one gets good sleep when they are in their own personal sauna. In addition, the change in hormones affects anxiety levels and depression. When you are anxious, you struggle to go to sleep and stay asleep.

Depression can result in a non-restful type of sleep. This can lead to a nasty cycle, as a lack of sleep can lead to anxiety and depression. Currie (2021) lists other ways that your decrease in hormones contributes to a lack of good sleep:

· Aches and pains in your joints

· Bladder issues – I get up at least two times a night to pee

· A decrease in progesterone can cause insomnia as it helps induce sleep

· Melatonin, the sleep hormone, decreases with age

<u>Sleep apnea</u>

According to Currie (2021), hot flashes and night sweats can contribute to sleep apnea. In addition, sleep apnea is associated with weight gain. A decrease in progesterone, which affects the muscle in the back of the neck, can also cause sleep apnea. Sleep apnea doesn't just manifest itself as loud snoring. It can also manifest as headaches, insomnia, daytime tiredness, depression, and anxiety. Wearing a mask may help you get the good night's sleep that you deserve.

<u>Restless leg syndrome</u>

If there was ever torture invented by the powers that be, it is restless leg syndrome. According to Currie (2021), women are twice as likely to experience restless leg syndrome than their male counterparts. The tingling, aching feeling in your legs at night, making it impossible to keep them still, is a sure bet that you won't get any sleep. One study suggests that almost seventy percent of women perceive the restless leg syndrome to be worse after they reached menopause.

Sleep hygiene

Having good sleep hygiene is one way that you can help beat insomnia. Currie (2021) describes several ways to practice good sleep hygiene.

<u>General</u>

1. It is important that you go to bed at a regular time – even on the weekends. When you get into a routine, your body knows it is time to sleep.

2. If you can, you should avoid taking naps during the day. If you feel as though you absolutely can't stay awake, don't sleep for more than thirty or forty minutes. Take your nap in the early afternoon – not in the late afternoon, and definitely not close to your bedtime.

3. Exercise on a regular basis. However, don't exercise within two hours of your bedtime. You aren't going to be able to do a workout with Richard Simmons and *Sweatin' to the Oldies* and then get to sleep an hour later.

4. Learn how much sleep you need to function. The average for most adults is six to eight hours a night, and this tends to decrease as you get older. However, your individual need for sleep might vary.

5. Make sure that you are taking your medication at the right time of day. For example, if your medication makes you drowsy, then it should be taken at night.

<u>Before you go to bed</u>

1. Our bodies love to operate on routines. You might

take a warm bath or read a book every night before you go to bed. Sticking to a routine helps your body know it's time to wind down and get ready for bed.

2. Try not to go to sleep if your belly is too full or if you are hungry. It's okay to have a light snack before you go to sleep. In the next section, we will talk about different types of foods that are great for inducing sleep.

3. Try to avoid drinking any caffeinated beverages for several hours before it's time to go to bed.

4. Although many people believe otherwise, alcohol does not induce a night of good sleep. Therefore, you should avoid drinking alcohol within a few hours before you hit the hay.

<u>Your sleeping environment</u>

1. Make sure that your bedroom has a cozy feel. It shouldn't be too cluttered with anything that will capture your attention and keep you awake.

2. Your bedroom should be cool. Getting a good night's rest when you're hot is almost impossible. However, your bedroom shouldn't be cold either. As Goldilocks would say, it needs to be just right.

3. Make sure your sheets, pillows, and mattress are comfortable.

4. Your bedroom should be used only for sleeping and sex. That way, when it's time to go into that room, your body automatically knows it is time to go to sleep.

5. Blue screens can affect your ability to sleep. You should avoid watching television or doing anything on

your phone, computer, or laptop for at least an hour before bed.

<u>If you wake up in the middle of the night</u>

1. If you can't go back to sleep within twenty minutes, get up and go into the other room. You aren't able to force yourself to sleep by staying in bed.

2. Once you get out of bed, do something quiet such as reading a book or coloring a picture in one of those fun coloring books.

3. It is important that whatever you do, you don't sit and watch the clock. The only thing you will accomplish is driving yourself up the wall. Also, avoid turning on the television.

4. Try not to think about your worries or problems while awake. We will talk about mindfulness later on in this chapter.

Food for sleeping

Do you remember all of those Thanksgiving and holiday dinners where people consumed turkey and then promptly fell asleep? That is because there is a protein in the turkey that induces sleep. There are several different types of food that you can eat before bedtime that can help you get the rest that you need. Registered dietician Brianna Elliott (2023) lists several foods you can try while trying to sleep.

<u>Almonds</u> -- Not only can almonds help you go to sleep, but they are also helpful in combatting the different health issues that are associated with the loss of estrogen. Eating

almonds on a regular basis has been shown to decrease different chronic diseases, such as type 2 diabetes and heart disease. It is high in healthy fats, fiber, and antioxidants.

Almonds will help you get to sleep and stay asleep because they are a good source of the sleep hormone melatonin. In addition, almonds are a good source of magnesium. One ounce of almonds accounts for nineteen percent of your daily recommended allowance. Magnesium helps decrease inflammation and reduce the stress hormone cortisol, which can cause insomnia.

<u>Turkey</u> -- Like almonds, turkey helps menopausal and postmenopausal in several ways. First, it is high in protein, which helps you maintain your muscle mass. It can help with weight gain, as turkey can help to regulate your appetite. Turkey helps you sleep because it contains the amino acid tryptophan. This helps increase your body's production of melatonin. Elliott (2023) states that the protein in turkey not only makes you tired so that you can fall asleep, but it also helps you wake up less during the night, which in turn, leads to a restful night's sleep.

<u>Chamomile tea</u> -- I'm sure the connection between chamomile tea and sleep is not new to you. The tea contains apigenin, which is an antioxidant. It binds itself to specific receptors in your brain that can make you sleepy. The tea can also help with some other issues associated with menopause. It contains flavones and antioxidants that decrease your risk of chronic diseases like cancer and heart disease. As a bonus, chamomile tea helps boost your

immune system. In addition, it can decrease anxiety and depression.

Kiwi – Elliot (2023) states that this low-calorie fruit is one of the best foods to eat before bed. She quotes one four-week study that indicated that adults who ate two kiwis an hour before bed could fall asleep forty-two percent faster than those who didn't eat anything before bed. The study indicated that their ability to sleep through the night increased by five percent. The participants' total sleep time increased by thirteen percent. Kiwis can help induce sleep because they are rich in serotonin, the hormone that, among other things, helps regulate your sleep cycle.

Tart cherry juice – The juice has high levels of magnesium and melatonin, which helps induce sleepiness and helps you stay asleep. Elliot (2023) cited one study in which adults suffering from insomnia drank two eight-ounce glasses of tart cherry juice each day for two weeks. The results were that they slept approximately eighty-four minutes longer than they had been. On top of that, their quality of sleep had improved.

Fatty fish – Fatty fish is a great food for many reasons. First, it can help you sleep better because they are high in vitamin D and omega-3 fatty acids. Together, these elements help increase your production of serotonin. Eating just a couple of ounces of fish before bed can help you get a good night's rest.

Fatty fish is good for menopausal and postmenopausal women in other ways. These fish are very rich in vitamin

D, which you will need to help your body process the calcium for healthy bones. The omega-3 fatty acids can reduce inflammation, which, in turn, helps protect you against heart disease. It also helps increase your brain health.

<u>Walnuts</u> – Like almonds and other tree nuts, walnuts are rich in magnesium and melatonin, which can help you fall asleep and stay asleep. Walnuts provide your body with alpha-linolenic acid and omega-3 fatty acids. Together they contribute to the production of serotonin.

They can reduce cholesterol levels, which contributes to heart disease. They are rich in healthy fats. Eating a handful of walnuts can also help reduce your appetite.

<u>Passionflower tea</u> – Like chamomile tea, passionflower tea has apigenin, which helps reduce anxiety. It has a calming effect on your brain, which is conducive to sleep. In addition, passionflower tea increases your brain's production of the GABA, inhibiting other chemicals that induce stress.

This tea has other benefits as well. It is rich in flavonoid antioxidants, reducing inflammation that can lead to heart disease. It also helps to boost your immunity.

<u>Dairy</u> – Cheese, milk, yogurt, and other dairy products are a source of the protein tryptophan, which is the same protein in turkeys that helps you sleep. Elliot (2023) states that milk has been shown to help adults sleep better

<u>Bananas</u> – Bananas contain magnesium, which helps to induce sleep.

<u>Oatmeal</u> – Oats are a source of melatonin. They are

high in carbs and are known to induce drowsiness when consumed right before bed.

HRT

Currie (2021) stated that hormone replacement therapy can help you sleep better. This is due, in part, because it treats hot flashes and night sweats. Studies have shown that when progesterone is part of the therapy, women have increased REM 3 sleep, where you get your most beneficial sleep.

Other medications

Your doctor may prescribe other types of medications to help treat your insomnia. These might include gabapentin and clonidine, which are antidepressants. Not only will they help treat your hot flashes and night sweats, but they can also decrease your anxiety and depression, which can play a role in insomnia.

Melatonin

Since your body's melatonin production decreases with age, your doctor may recommend a melatonin supplement. Make sure that you talk to your doctor before starting any supplements.

Mindfulness

One important tool that you can use to help you deal with some of your symptoms is mindfulness. According to the Mayo Clinic (2019), women who practice mindfulness may experience fewer menopausal symptoms. This is especially true if you are experiencing anxiety, depression, or irritability. A study of more than seventeen hundred menopausal and postmenopausal women indicated that those who practiced mindfulness experienced fewer symptoms.

It is a good tool to use when you are trying to sleep at night, and your brain chooses to go over every single mistake you've ever made or go into detail about all the chores on your to-do list for the next thirty years.

Practicing mindfulness means that you focus your thoughts on the here and now. You aren't worried about the past or what will happen in twenty minutes, tomorrow, or whenever. The easiest way to practice mindfulness is to focus on your breathing. Pay attention to the rise and fall of your chest. Feel the air as you breathe in through your nose and then out through your mouth.

At some point, you will notice that your mind has wandered. *I'm not thinking about breathing. I'm considering that I have to do a million chores.* Just return your thoughts to your breathing and continue. (Hoshaw, 2022).

There are other ways to practice mindfulness. For example, if you are using mindfulness while walking, you focus on the sound of your foot hitting the ground and how it feels to take each step. You concentrate on the sounds going on around you as you walk. Smell the air (Howshaw, 2022).

You can practice mindfulness on every task you undertake, focusing on your senses as you work. For example, I can focus on the sounds of my keyboard and my dog snoring. I smell the lemon from my diffuser and hear the TV in the next room.

In addition to helping decrease menopausal symptoms, mindfulness can help you in many other ways (Howshaw, 2022). It can decrease anxiety and depression as you purposefully turn your thoughts away from those causing stress. It can help you sleep as you ask your mind to think about how comfortable your bed is, how the sheets feel, etc. Mindful eating can help you lose weight. Use mindfulness to guide your thoughts away from the joint and muscle aches and pain that accompany menopause to help decrease your discomfort.

One of the great advantages of mindfulness is that it can help you with motivation, concentration, and focus. I've noticed that since I hit menopause (or it hit me), my motivation has decreased. In the past, I have been very enthusiastic about writing my day's to-do list and tackling it. Now, I look at it, and I'm like eh. Even when I try to get the work done, I struggle to focus. My mind wanders everywhere. However, I can use mindfulness to help alleviate these problems. I pick one task. I decide what I need to do to get it done, and take the first step. When my focus starts to wander, I recognize that my thoughts have moved somewhere else, and then I purposefully move my brain back to the task at hand. It feels good to cross that task off once it's accomplished.

Psychotherapy

Cognitive behavioral therapy (CBT) can be helpful as you try to find different ways to deal with the symptoms of menopause. Hunter and Smith (2023) say that CBT can help teach you new ways to manage problems. It can help you learn new coping skills and strategies to handle the symptoms.

Research has shown that menopause can increase our anxiety and depression because of the decreased levels of estrogen. On top of that, menopause usually happens at a time in our lives when we are dealing with other outside issues that contribute to our anxiety levels, such as taking care of elderly parents and children who are leaving the nest. Hunter and Smith (2023) state that the anxiety and stress we feel can lead to heart palpitations and hot flashes, especially if we are prone to anxiety attacks. Our stressful thoughts can also prevent us from getting a good night's rest or lead to overeating. Cognitive behavioral therapy can help decrease those feelings.

Cognitive behavioral therapy can teach you how to overcome the negative thoughts that cause hot flashes, insomnia, headaches, etc. For example, Hunger and Smith (2023) state that a lot of women see the arrival of menopause as the time when they are getting old. They start to feel as though they look old, and wrinkles appear. It is important to ask yourself if it is really the truth or if you are the same person you've always been. You can exchange stressful thoughts with more helpful thoughts.

Another example that Hunter and Smith (2023) give is about hot flashes. Instead of being upset about them, you can tell yourself, "I handled the last hot flashes like a pro. I can handle this flash just fine." Instead of thinking that the hot flash lasts forever, you can tell yourself it will go away like the last one. Exchanging negative thoughts with more positive ones can make the experiences less intense.

On top of being beneficial in helping you sleep better, regulate your eating to help control your weight, and help make your hot flashes less intense, it can also help you decrease your chances for heart disease. When you are stressed out, your body produces more of the stress hormone, cortisol. When your body constantly has high levels of cortisol, blood pressure increases, as does your chances of heart disease.

Hypnosis

Research has shown that hypnotherapy is another tool that can mitigate some of the symptoms of menopause (Jack, 2020). It can help reduce the frequency and severity of those personal summers. It can also help decrease your depression and anxiety levels. According to Dr. Clair Jack (2020), women who focused on cooling imagery in a hypnotic state had more control over their hot flashes and night sweats. In some cases, the women were even able to prevent them. The research indicated that hypnosis was as effective as hormone replacement therapy as it reduced approximately seventy-four percent of hot flashes and night sweats.

Jack (2020) gave three ways to use hypnotic techniques to help decrease the frequency and intensity of hot flashes and anxiety levels.

<u>Cool imagery</u> – Jack (2020) states that you should take some time to get into a relaxed state. You can use the

relaxed state you are in when you meditate, or you can imagine breathing in a cool, silvery light through your nostrils and letting that light flow through your body as you exhale. As you tell yourself you are becoming increasingly relaxed, you will continue to envision this. Once you are very relaxed, you can picture the most cooling situation you can think of, such as swimming in a pool or being outside where a cool breeze is flowing around you. Focus on this image with everything that you have. Then, you can focus on this image the next time you experience a hot flash or night sweats.

<u>Your future self</u> – Jones (2020) states that you should concentrate on how you would like to feel six months from now. You should close your eyes and picture as many details as possible. Use your senses to see what is going on around you. Pay attention to what you will smell and what you will hear. Think about how you will be feeling. Then, figure out what steps you need to take to get to this point. This may include lifestyle changes, incorporating some meditation or yoga techniques, or other methods. The more you focus on this image of yourself the more real it will be come.

<u>Flash control dial</u> – You will imagine you are in a room for this technique. A dial on one of the walls ranges from zero to ten. Zero represents you feeling comfortable and cool. Ten represents feeling very hot like you would during a hot flash. Close your eyes and picture what you are feeling between zero and ten. Turn up the dial so you feel very hot, and hold it there for a few seconds. Then, turn the dial back

down so that you are comfortable. If you practice this before you start to have hot flashes, you can easily turn down the dial when experiencing one.

Cool Hot Flashes

Hot flashes are one of the two things that really make my life difficult. However, there are ways you can help decrease the severity of your personal summers, short of stripping off your clothes and jumping in an ice-cold bathtub.

Hunter and Smith (2023) advised wearing layers of light clothing to take off when the hot flashes hit and put back on when the chills take over. You should wear loose-fitting cotton clothes. You can also carry a small portable fan with you. To help with the night sweats, you should have lower thread count cotton sheets. Hunter and Smith (2023) state that a Chillow Pillow can also help you stay cool at night.

You should focus on relaxing when the hot flashes or night sweats hit. Hunter and Smith (2023) say that our threshold for temperature decreases if we are stressed out and anxious about them. Instead of letting your mind concentrate on how miserable you are at the moment, you should pace your breathing and focus on that.

Support groups

The most important thing I can tell you is that you are not alone. There are millions of women in the world who are going through what you are. It is easier to deal with the symptoms when we know that someone in our corner is going through the same experiences. It also helps when you can share tips on handling the different emotions and physical symptoms brought on by menopause. Support groups are a great tool for that. Check out one below:

Red Hot Mamas: https://www.inspire.com/groups/red-hot-mamas-menopause/

Menopause and Me: https://www.menopause.org/for-women

Hormones Health and Healing: https://www.meetup.com/hormones-health-and-healing/

Menopause Matters: https://www.menopausematters.co.uk/forum/index.php

Menopause ChitChat: https://forum.menopause-chitchat.com

Menopause Café: https://www.menopausecafe.net

Conclusion

Menopause has arrived and brought with it all kinds of not so fun symptoms. However, you don't have to suffer in silence. You don't have to suffer at all. There are so many ways that you can help to overcome them. This chapter discussed several methods you can use to deal with insomnia, hot flashes, anxiety, depression, and even the more frightening prospects of cancer and heart disease.

Right now, I would like you to take a minute to practice mindfulness. Get comfortable (but not so comfortable that you fall asleep). I want you to think about your breathing. Concentrate on how it feels to breathe in the air and then breathe it out. When another thought intrudes, recognize it and gently push it away as you focus on your breathing. Practicing this technique will make it easier to use the next time you have a hot flash or can't sleep.

How do you feel? Note the techniques you want to use to help you thrive during this time so you're not at the mercy of your symptoms. When you're ready, we'll move on to chapter six, discussing different physical techniques you can use to combat your menopausal symptoms.

Chapter 6

Meditation, Yoga, Acupuncture, and other Stress-Relieving Techniques to Help You on Your Menopausal Journey

"There is something wonderfully bold and liberating about saying yes to our entire imperfect and messy life." ~ Tara Brach

My husband loves to go to Lowes and Home Depot, browsing through the tool section. Each time, he finds something that he needs. I asked him why he needed another tool since he already had some that would do the job. He always tells me that it is important to have the right tools needed to get the job done even better. There is no such thing as too many tools.

The same idea works for finding the best way to deal with menopausal symptoms. Sometimes, one tool works better than the other, and sometimes you might use a combination of several tools to get the job done. In that spirit, we will discuss some additional tools you can use, alone or in addition to others, to help you live a comfortable and healthy life.

Meditation

Some studies have indicated that meditation can help reduce some of the symptoms of menopause. You can use meditation techniques to reduce the frequency and severity of hot flashes and night sweats. One study showed that women who suffered from at least seven moderate to severe hot flashes a day indicated that after they practiced guided meditation for at least forty-five minutes six days a week, the frequency of their hot flashes decreased by thirty-nine percent. The severity of their hot flashes decreased by forty percent (WebMD, 2006).

In addition, meditation relieves stress, which means that it can help reduce anxiety and depression. Many research studies have shown that meditating for at least ten minutes each day will lower your cholesterol and blood pressure, decreasing your risks of heart disease, type 2 diabetes, and strokes (Providence, 2021). Not only will your risks of these disease decrease, but since you are less stressed out, you can sleep better.

Getting started

Sometimes, the most challenging part of any activity is figuring out how to get started. Meditation is no different. However, life trainer, Babauta (n.d.) has twenty tips that you can use to get started.

1. Start small. Babauta (n.d.) suggests that you sit still for two minutes every day for a week. After a week, add another

couple of minutes to your daily routine. Before you know it, you will meditate for ten minutes daily.

2. Meditate first thing in the morning so you don't get so busy that you run out of time or simply forget. Make sure you leave a reminder somewhere so that you know you are supposed to meditate before you start your day.

3. Don't worry about how you are supposed to meditate. Just make a plan to do it. Don't worry about how or where you are supposed to sit. Just sit where you are comfortable. You are only meditating for two minutes at a time initially, so how and where you sit isn't relevant. Later on, when you meditate for longer periods, you can figure out what position is most comfortable (Babauta, n.d.).

4. Babauta (n.d). said that you should check in with yourself when you first start to meditate. Think about how you feel emotionally and physically. He said realizing that whatever feelings you are "bringing to the meditation session" are acceptable is important.

5. Once you have started to get the hang of making time to meditate, then you should count your breaths. While you are sitting, focus your attention on your breathing. Pay attention to the air as you breathe it in, and follow the journey it takes as it makes its way to your lungs. Count your breaths. Count one as you breathe in and two as you breathe out. Count to ten and then start over again.

6. Know that your mind will wander. When it does, just acknowledge it and return to your breathing, starting with the count of one.

7. Don't judge your thoughts and feelings when you meditate. Babauta (n.d.) states that it is important to look at them as friends, as they are a part of who you are – not all of who you are.

8. Don't worry about whether you are doing it wrong. There is no perfect way to meditate. It is important to be pleased that you are simply meditating.

9. You shouldn't worry about clearing your mind. Babauta (n.d) states that many people believe that meditation means that you have to clear your mind or stop all of your thoughts. Instead, practice focusing your thoughts or attention, such as breathing.

10. Once you have practiced meditation for a while and have worked on returning your thoughts to your breathing, you can start practicing staying with your thoughts when your mind wanders. If you are feeling anxiety, sadness, or whatever, you can stay with the thought and "be curious." It is important that you don't judge your thoughts and feelings. Accept them.

11. Meditation is about getting to know yourself and understanding how your brain works. Observing how your mind wanders, avoids negative feelings, and even gets frustrated can help you learn about yourself.

12. Treat yourself with kindness, and as you get to know yourself, do it as though you are learning about a friend.

13. You can do a body scan once you focus on your breath. Start at your feet. Focus on the soles of your feet and ask yourself how they feel. Then move to your toes and the

tops of your feet. Keep moving until you reach the top of your head.

14. Pay attention to the light, sounds, and energy around you. Once you have practiced counting your breathing, you can also focus on the room's light, sound and energy while keeping your eyes in one spot.

15. Commit yourself to meditate for at least a month.

16. Remember that you can meditate anywhere. Although Babauta (n.d.) says that meditating while sitting is best, you can meditate while walking, standing, or in any position. You can also meditate anywhere, whether you are in your office, commuting to work, or taking a walk.

17. Try guided meditation if it works. We will discuss guided meditation in the next section.

18. Check in with other people. Even if you choose to meditate alone, you can check in with friends and family and let them know that you did meditate for the day. The accountability will mean that you are more likely to stick to your routine.

19. Join a community of people who meditate.

20. Smile when you have finished your first two minutes. Celebrate that you had that time for yourself, that you stuck with it, and that you took the time to get to know yourself better.

Guided meditations

Everyone approaches meditation differently. For some, especially beginners, guided meditations can be very helpful. Guided meditations are when a meditation expert guides you into a meditative state. You focus on what the expert is saying and envision it. One of my favorite guided meditations is when the man describes a nice blue sky with a fluffy cloud. Then, I picture myself enveloped in one of those clouds, floating along, leaving all my stress behind. I focus a hundred percent of my attention on what it feels like to be in that cloud. The only problem is that I get so relaxed that sometimes I fall asleep. That is why I always have a timer to alert me when my time is up.

Everheart (2023), a meditation instructor, provides tips to get the most out of your sessions.

First, you will want to find a comfortable relaxing place with minimal distractions. She reminds you not to get so comfortable that you fall asleep.

Second, listen to the person talking and lightly follow the instructions. You don't need to concentrate hard on what is being said.

Third, don't try to get rid of intrusive thoughts. Instead, acknowledge them and return your attention to the voice.

Fourth, don't have expectations. There is no right or wrong way to meditate, but if you have certain expectations on how it should go, you will be disappointed—and lastly, practice. The more you practice guided meditation, the more you will see the results you are hoping for.

Everheart (2023) states that you can do guided meditations whenever needed. If you are anxious and stressed out at work, you can sit in your car during your break and meditate. You can also choose to start or end your day with guided meditations. Since you can download guided meditations on your phone and practice them anywhere.

Depending on your goals, you can use guided meditations as a quick fix to a stressful situation or when you simply feel the need. There are also technique-based guided meditations if you have long-term goals (Everheart, 2023).

Word repetition

The North American Menopause Society (NAMS)) describes one type of meditation that can be useful when you start to experience hot flashes or you are feeling stress or anxiety (n.d.).

1. To start, pick a particular word or phrase that you are comfortable repeating.

2. Find a comfortable, quiet place to sit.

3. Relax your body, starting with your feet and moving to your head and neck.

4. Breathe naturally, focusing on your word or phrase as you exhale.

5. If your mind begins to wander, acknowledge it, then return your focus to your breathing and word or phrase.

6. Practice this between ten and twenty minutes at least once a day.

Paced breathing

The NAMS (n.d.) recommends paced breathing as a great way to help with hot flashes.

1. Sit straight in a chair with both feet flat on the floor.

2. Rest your hands on your abdomen.

3. Count to four slowly as you breathe in through your nose. Feel your abdomen rising as you inhale.

4. Hold that breath in for a second.

5. Exhale through your mouth to the slow count of four while feeling your abdomen falling.

6. Practice this exercise twice daily for fifteen minutes or when you feel a hot flash coming on.

Guided muscle relaxation:

When you get stressed out and feel anxious, your body tenses up. One technique you can use to release that tension is the guided muscle relaxation technique. Not only does it help at the moment, but practicing this technique over time can decrease your stress and anxiety levels (Saranchock, 2023), decreasing your blood pressure.

You will work on relaxing your muscles one step at a time. Saranchock (2023) states that you should skip that particular step if you have an injury or pain in any area. He also emphasizes that as you go through the different steps and tense the muscles in that particular group, you shouldn't overdo it to the point where your muscles start to cramp, strain, or hurt.

1. The first step is to get into a comfortable position. You might be more comfortable lying on the couch or floor or sitting upright. Close your eyes. Then, you should breathe deeply. Breathe in slowly and out slowly. After you've taken a couple of breaths, imagine that any tension you are feeling is released when you exhale. Continue to relax as you breathe deeply.

2. Start with your right hand and forearm. Make a tight fist and then bend your fist back at your wrist. Feel the tension. Hold that pose for five seconds and then relax your fist and wrist, noticing the release of tension.

3. Bend your right arm and tense it like you are showing off your muscles. Tighten your bicep as much as possible. Hold it for five seconds, then let your arm go limp as you breathe.

4. Repeat these actions with your left hand, wrist, and arm. Hold the tense pose for five seconds, then breathe as you release them.

5. Move onto your forehead next. Wrinkle your forehead as tightly as you can. Raise your eyebrows as high as possible. After five seconds, release the tension.

6. Your face is next. Make sure that your eyes are squeezed tightly shut and your cheeks tense. Release after five seconds, remembering to breathe deeply.

7. Open your mouth as wide as possible as though you are giving your most enormous yawn. Feel the tension release as you relax your jaw muscles after five seconds.

8. Tense your neck muscles next. Afterward, let your neck sink into whatever surface is available, completely relaxing.

9. Clench your shoulders tightly as you raise them to your ears. Then, after you count to five, lower and relax them. Notice how the tension has left your shoulders.

10. Breathe deeply, filling your lung as much as possible. Tense the muscles in your ribs and upper back. After five

seconds, release the air, picturing all your tension leaving your body as you exhale.

11. Focus on tightening your stomach while ensuring that all other muscles are as relaxed as possible. Notice how your stomach softens when you release the muscles.

12. The next step is to arch your back away from whatever surface you're on. While you are squeezing your shoulder blades you tense the muscles in your lower back. Then, loosen your muscles and let your back sink back into whatever surface you are on.

13. Squeeze your glutes together tightly for five seconds. Then, release the muscles.

14. Tighten your right thigh holding it if five seconds, feeling the tension from your hip to your knee. Then, loosen the muscles, feeling the tension leave. Repeat with your left thigh. You can lift your knee a little if it helps.

15. Tighten your right calf, holding that muscle tight for five seconds before releasing it. Repeat with your left calf.

16. Turn your attention to your right foot. Slowly curl your toes toward your foot, tightly tensing your foot for five seconds before relaxing. Repeat with your left foot.

17. Now, turn your attention to your entire body. Feel your entire body relaxing from the top of your head to the soles of your feet. Continue to breathe deeply and slowly as you feel the tension flowing out of you. Feel your belly rising and falling with deep breaths, and slowly open your eyes. Stay still for a few minutes until your body is alert and ready to go on with your day.

Sensory grounding

Ashley Abramson (2023), who has written extensively on health issues, including menopausal health, suggests sensory grounding. You can use this meditation technique whenever and wherever you need to. It is beneficial when you are stressed or starting to experience a hot flash. By focusing all your attention on what one of your senses detects, you can push out the negative thoughts and feelings.

Sit with your back straight up. Put your hands on your legs with your palms up. Then, close your eyes.

Choose one of your senses. For example, concentrate on everything that you can smell. You might detect a hint of your co-worker's aftershave. Perhaps you can smell the coffee from the coffee pot. If you're outside, you might smell the flowers around you, fresh-cut grass, and the pond that is close by. If a thought tries to intrude, acknowledge it and then put all of your attention back on what you are smelling.

After a couple of minutes, once your tension has decreased, you can open your eyes and return to your tasks.

Loving-kindness meditation:

When we are struggling or stressed out, we are hard on ourselves. However, a lot of research indicates that you will be able to deal with stress or anxiety if you practice self-compassion (Abramson, 2022). Loving-kindness meditation can help you have more compassion toward yourself and lead to more positive thinking.

First, you should find a quiet, comfortable place to sit.

Put your hand on your chest. Then, you simply start saying kind phrases to yourself. You might say phrases telling yourself that you can get through a rough patch in your life. "I can get through this stressful time." You might also focus on desires or feelings. "I deserve to feel calmness and peace." If it helps, you can picture people who care about you hugging you as you state the affirmations (Abramson, 2022).

Bedtime meditations

Insomnia is my most dreaded symptom of menopause. When I can't get enough sleep, all the other symptoms hit me tenfold. I can't concentrate on any of my tasks. Abramson (2022) recommends a bedtime meditation.

When you are ready to sleep, lay in bed and close your eyes. Focus on letting your body relax and staying still. Then, shift your thoughts to your breathing. Take deep breaths in through your nose and then let them out through your mouth. As you breathe in, focus your attention on the air. Visualize it as it goes to your lungs, and then travel with it as it moves through your body – into your brain, face, hands, feet, and back out. As you exhale, imagine all your tension and stress are leaving the body. As you breathe in the air, picture it as a life force or as energizing your body. When you exhale, your breath removes all toxins from your body (Abramson, 2022).

Yoga

Yoga instructor, Patricia Walden, was suffering from all the symptoms that accompanied menopause. She would wake up in the middle of the night and not be able to get back to sleep for several hours. She suffered from fatigue and hot flashes. She had been doing a regular yoga routine each day but discovered that not only were the routines not helping her symptoms, but they were actually making them worse. So, she turned to routines that helped relieve stress and anxiety without aggravating hot flashes (Gura, 2019).

Yoga poses designed to decrease severity and intensity of hot flashes

Because physical tension of your body can make your hot flashes worse, Walden recommends that you engage in restorative poses. There are several that can help decrease the severity and intensity of hot flashes. Examples of restorative poses include the happy baby pose and the child's pose.

<u>Happy baby pose</u>

The happy baby pose is designed to help you focus on flexibility, strength, and breathing. The goal of this restorative pose is to promote mental well-being. It is often recommended for beginners (Higuera, 2020). She offers the following instructions on how to correctly do the happy baby pose.

1. Lie flat on your back.

2. Keeping your head down, bring your knees toward your chest so they are at a ninety-degree angle. The soles of your feet should be faced toward the ceiling.

3. Reach up to grab either the insides or the outsides of your feet. Move your knees apart toward your armpits.

4. Flex your heels and rock side to side gently, as a happy

baby would do. Stay in this position as you inhale and exhale deeply several times.

<u>Child's pose</u>

Pizer (2020), a registered yoga instructor, says that this beginner pose is the most important resting pose in yoga. The child's pose is great for stretching your back, hips, thighs, and ankles. This pose can help alleviate your back pain as well. Pizer (2020) provides the following instructions:

1. Get on your hands and knees on your mat.

2. With your feet on the mat and your big toes touching, spread your knees so that they are as wide as your mat.

3. Let your belly rest between your thighs. Rest your forehead on the floor. Relax your face and your shoulders. If you can't rest your forehead comfortably on the floor, you can rest it on a block or on your fists. This is important because "There is an energy point at the center of the fore-head in between the eyebrows that stimulates the vagus nerve and supports a 'rest and digest' response. Finding a comfortable place for the forehead is key to gaining this soothing benefit," (Pizer, 2020).

4. There are several different ways that you can rest your arms. One variation is for you to stretch out your arms in front of you, palms down. You can also stretch your arms back, next to your thighs, with the palms down. Or you can stretch your arms forward with your palms up. Pizer (2020) also suggests that you could bend your elbows and let your thumbs rest on your neck.

5. Focus on your breathing as you stay in this position for as long as you want to.

Patricia Walden also recommends that you use different props, such as bolsters, or blankets to help support you as you engage in the different poses. Walden states that putting your head on a chair or bolster while you are doing a forward bend can help relax your nerves and calm your brain. Reclining poses that are supported can also help you achieve complete relaxation. She recommends three different reclining poses that can help provide relief from hot flashes. These are the reclining bound pose, reclining hero pose, and half plow pose (Gura, 2019).

<u>Reclining bound pose</u>

This pose is also known as the reclined cobbler's pose. There are many benefits of this pose in addition to helping to alleviate the severity and frequency of hot flashes. Everyday Yoga (2015) states that it can, among other things, decrease your blood pressure, heart rate, and frequency of headaches, and help relieve insomnia and fatigue. It can alleviate stress, tension, and anxiety – all symptoms associated with menopause. Everyday Yoga (2015) explains the following steps of how to successfully do this pose.

1. You will sit on your mat with your back straight up and down, your legs straight out in front of you, and your hands, palms down, resting next to your hips. Then, you should bend your knees, pulling your heels in toward your pelvic bone. The soles of your feet should be pressed together as you let your knees drop open on each side.

2. Lean backward so that your head touches the floor, or on a block if you need the added support. Bring your elbows down to the floor.

3. Move your glutes from side to side. This will help you adjust your position while lengthening your spine along the floor while keeping the natural curve of your back intact.

4. Pull your shoulders in while letting your arms relax. Keep your palms up.

5. Allow your glutes to relax and let your pelvic lengthen toward your feet.

6. Close your eyes and focus your attention internally.

7. Breathe naturally. As you maintain this pose, let your body start to feel heavy.

8. Stay in this position for one to ten minutes.

<u>Reclining hero pose</u>

Pizer (2021) states that there are many benefits to this pose, including the fact that it can help decrease lower back pain and improve blood circulation. She provides instructions on how to do this pose:

1. You will start with the hero pose, which means that you are sitting with your back straight. Your legs are bent at the knees so that your feet are on either side of your hips.

2. Put your hands on either side of your hips. Then, as you lean back, walk your hands back toward your glutes.

3. Bend your arms so that you are leaning on your forearms. If you are leaning on a block then you won't take this pose any further.

4. If you are comfortable leaning on your elbows, you

can continue leaning backward until your back reaches the floor. However, if you start to feel any pain, then you may have leaned too far back. You should go back to leaning on your forearms.

5. Keep your knees together during this process.

6. Stay in the position for approximately five to ten breaths.

<u>Half plow pose</u>

The half plow pose, in addition to relieving hot flashes, can help relieve back aches. It stretches several muscles, such as your shoulders, back, and neck. Pizer (2021) gives the instructions for the half plow pose.

1. Lie on your back.

2. Lay your arms on the ground, extending them forward with your palms down.

3. Using your palms and forearms for leverage, bring your legs up to ninety degrees.

4. Stay in this position for five to ten breaths.

Yoga poses for memory

As I mentioned, I have been known to walk into a room and then immediately forget why I'm there. This is because of the hormone fluctuations that happen during menopause. Memory issues can become a lot worse if you are struggling to get enough rest at night or are feeling anxious. Walden states that the same poses that help to counteract depression can also help you deal with your frag-mented thoughts. She mentioned the downward facing dog position and the corpse pose (Gura, 2019).

. . .

Downward facing dog pose

In addition to helping you with your memory issues, the downward facing dog pose works to stretch several of your muscles, such as your calves and hamstrings. Pizer (2021) provides step-by-step instructions for the pose.

1. Get down on your hands and knees. Your wrists should be under your shoulders and your knees should be under your hips.

2. Curl your toes. Then, you should push with your hands so that your hips are lifted, and your legs are straight.

3. Spread your fingers. Then, push down from your forearms into your fingertips.

4. Rotate your upper arms outwardly to broaden your collarbones.

5. Allow your head to hang down. Push your shoulders toward your hips.

6. Your leg muscles, or quadriceps, should bear the bulk of the weight. This takes the majority of the weight off of your arms.

7. You should then move your thighs inward. Make sure that your butt is in the air. Press your heels into the ground.

8. Exhale and then move back to your hands and knees by bending your legs.

Corpse pose

The corpse pose is a resting pose that is often used after a yoga session. While you are in this pose, you should be reflecting on what you've experienced during your session. It should help you wind down after your workout and relax. This is also a useful pose to practice right before you go to sleep since the goal of this pose is to quiet your mind. Pizer (2022) tells us how to do this pose.

1. Lay down, flat on your back.

2. Move your legs so that they are not touching. Let your feet fall to the side.

3. Your arms should be next to your body, but not touching you. Your palms should be up. Allow your fingers to curl.

4. Your shoulder blades should be tucked onto your back to provide support.

5. Relax your entire body -- your face included. Allow your body to feel heavy.

6. Breathe naturally. Focus on your breathing. If your mind starts to wander, bring it gently back to your breathing.

7. You should stay in this position for five to ten minutes.

Yoga for fatigue

Fatigue was one of the worst symptoms for me. I just always felt so tired all of the time. I didn't even want to do my favorite activities. Walden suggests that yoga poses that use backbends can be very beneficial. Not only does it help you feel safe and nourished, it opens your chest so that your breathing and circulation are improved. Walden recommends reclined goddess pose (Gura, 2019).

<u>Reclined goddess pose</u>

Pizer (2020) says that this particular pose helps to quiet your mind. It also helps to open up your groin area and your hips. It can help stretch the hip flexors, which can be beneficial if you sit a lot. This pose can also help relieve back pain and sciatica. Pizer (2020) explains how to do this pose.

1. Lie down on your back.

2. Bend your knees while keeping your feet flat on the floor.

3. Open your knees as you bring the bottoms of your feet together.

4. Allow your arms to be in any position that is comfortable.

5. You should stay in this pose for several minutes, allowing gravity to help deepen the stretch. Breathe naturally while you are in this pose.

Yoga to help you deal with irritability, insomnia, and anxiety

Spikes in your estrogen levels or sharp declines in your progesterone levels can cause you to feel anxious, nervous, or irritable. This will increase your heart rate, as well as other symptoms. Prolonged stress only makes these symptoms worse. According to Walden, forward bends can decrease stress and irritability because they help you push away external distractions, which in turn, helps soothe your mind. The poses can also help with insomnia because the poses ground your energy and help to alleviate anxiety. If you follow the bends with restorative postures, such as the corpse pose, it can help you achieve a deep, restive sleep. Walden recommends the standing forward bend and the wide-legged forward bend (Gura, 2019).

<u>Standing forward bend</u>

In addition to helping you deal with the irritability, insomnia, and anxiety that accompanies menopause, the standing forward bend helps you stretch your hamstrings and calves. Pizer (2022) explains how to do this bend. Start with the mountain pose described in steps 1 – 10 (Pizer, 2022).

1. For this pose your big toes will touch as you stand straight. Then, you will lift your toes off the floor and stretch them out before putting your feet back on the ground. You can separate your heels if your ankles are touching.

2. Allow your calves and feet to press into the ground.

3. Use your front thigh muscles to engage, which will pull your kneecaps up.

4. Rotate your thighs so that they are facing inward, which will widen your sit bones, or your lower pelvis. These are the bones that bear your weight when you sit.

5. Your back should stay in its natural curve.

6. Suck in your belly, slightly.

7. Make sure that your shoulders are over your pelvis. Spread your collarbones.

8. Draw your shoulders up to your ears. Then you should roll them back.

9. Your arms should be hanging by your side. There

should be a slight bend in your elbows and your palms should face forward.

10. Your neck should be long with your chin straight forward. The top of your head should be toward the ceiling.

For the next part of this pose, you will move from the mountain pose to the raised hands pose as described in steps 11 – 14 (Pizer, 2022).

11. Inhale while you are moving your arms out from your sides and toward the sky.

12. You should bring your palms together over your head if you can without hunching your shoulders. If you can't, and your hands aren't touching, then the palms of your hands should face each other. Your arms should be straight. Look up toward your thumbs.

13. Move your shoulders back from your ears as you broaden your collar bones. If it feels as though your ribs are pulling apart then move so they are together. Make sure that your quads are still pulling your kneecaps up.

14. While your hands are over your head, press your feet into the ground as you lift the top of your head. Pull your belly button in toward your spine while making sure that your sternum is lifted.

After you are in the raised hand pose, you will move into the standing forward bend as described by Pizer (2022).

15. Your arms should sweep down to be in a forward fold in front of your hips. This motion is usually referred to as the swan dive.

16. Then, you will put your hands on the mat, palms

down. Pizer (2022) suggests using blocks if your hands don't reach the floor.

17. Bend your knees just a tiny bit to ensure they aren't locked.

18. Make sure that your quads are engaged and draw them up. This will help open up the muscles in the back of your thighs or the hamstrings.

19. Put your weight on the balls of your feet so that your hips are over your ankles.

20. Allow your head to hang down.

21. Come out of the pose as you inhale, pushing your pelvis down and using your abs.

<u>Wide-legged forward bend</u>

Yoga Basics (2023) describes how to do this particular pose.

1. Start with the mountain pose. Then, you will move your legs about three or four feet apart. This is the five-pointed star. Exhale as you press your palms to the mat under your shoulders.

2. Pull your forehead toward the floor. Your elbows will bend toward the wall behind you. Put the weight on your feet as you lengthen your legs, pushing your hips toward the ceiling.

3. Feel your spine stretch as your head is down and your hips are up.

4. Hold this pose for three to eight breaths.

5. Move back into the five-pointed star as you inhale.

· · ·

Yoga for depression and mood swings

Menopause often comes with bouts of depression. This can be because your progesterone levels increase or your estrogen levels decrease. However, yoga has been known to help alter moods. Walden states that backbends, especially when they are done using supports, can "allow a sense of lightness into the body" (Gura, 2019). It also stimulates your adrenal glands, as well as expands your chest so that you can breathe in more oxygen. Walden suggests the shoulder stand to help combat depression (Gura, 2019).

<u>Shoulder stand</u>

Pizer (2021) suggests that you use folded blankets as support when you do this pose. The blankets should be lined up with the end of your mat. She explains how to do the pose with the following steps.

1. You start off with your shoulders and upper back on the blankets while your head and neck are off the blankets. Your legs should be bent and your feet should be on the floor. You should move your shoulders so they are under your upper back. You will feel your chest rise a bit.

2. Lift your hips off the mat while you are extending your arms out on the mat. Your palms should be facing down.

3. Use your palms to help you move onto the balls of your feet, and then extend one of your legs up into the air.

4. Bend your arms and put your hands on your lower back and then extend your other leg up into the air. Make sure that you are looking up and that your neck is straight.

5. Walk your hands further up your back. You should feel your chest reach toward your chin, with your upper back being supported.

6. Your hips should move toward the front while your feet are pointed toward the back so that your body is straight. The correct alignment for this position is for your hips to be over your shoulders and your feet to be over your hips.

7. Stay in this pose for about ten breaths.

Practicing yoga

These are just a few of the different poses that can help you combat your menopausal symptoms. There are many advantages of practicing yoga. There are a lot of different poses that are good for beginners. Then, as you practice, you can learn more difficult poses. You can practice yoga practically anywhere at any time. If you choose, you can practice yoga on your own or you can join a studio. However you go about it, you will reap the benefits of yoga.

Acupuncture

Although the thought of needles being put into certain pressure points to access parts of our brain may sound frightening, it is a very ancient type of medicine and has proven benefits. One study showed that after undergoing acupuncture medicine for five weeks, the participants had decreased the incidents of hot flashes and night sweats. Their mood swings eased as did their insomnia, as well as fatigue, anxiety, pain, and vaginal dryness. The researchers stated that acupuncture was a safe treatment that wasn't too costly. There were very few side effects of the treatment (Bringle, 2021).

How does acupuncture work?

The acupuncturist inserts tiny needles through your skin at different points of your body. It is based on the theory of ying and yang, where your life force or energy in your body has to stay balanced in order for you to be healthy. It is believed that this life force flows through your body a certain way. The needles are placed in strategic points, along the pathways or meridians, to make sure that your life force stays balanced (Mayo Clinic, 2023).

How does acupuncture feel?

Hair-thin needles are used during acupuncture. Because they are so tiny, most people report that they do not feel any pain or just slight pain during the procedure. When the needles are inserted, you may feel slight pressure or an ache. Once they are inserted, the needles might be heated or have mild electricity applied to them. The practitioner may also twirl the needles. The needles usually stay in between ten and fifteen minutes. You shouldn't feel any pain when the needles are removed (John Hopkins, 2023).

Acupuncture to treat menopausal symptoms

<u>Hot flashes and night sweats</u>

In addition to staying hydrated, acupuncture helps to ensure that there is balance in the kidneys. It helps to make sure that there is no hormonal imbalance that would make your bodily temperatures rise (Bringle, 2021).

. . .

<u>Pain</u>

Acupuncture has been recommended by the American College of Physicians as a means of relieving lower back pain and aches associated with menopause. Inserting the needles at specific pressure points stimulates your central nervous system. This causes your brain to release chemicals, such as endorphins, that alleviate pain and aches (Bringle, 2021).

<u>Mood swings and anxiety</u>

One study, conducted in 2013, discovered that acupuncture can change the brain's neurotransmitters in such a way that it relieves anxiety and nervousness.

<u>Insomnia</u>

Acupuncture was shown to alleviate insomnia in a study conducted in 2019. Activating a pressure point that is just above your ankle, called the three yin intersection, can help relieve insomnia. Experts also suggest that soaking your feet, up to the three yin intersection, in hot water and Epsom salt can help you sleep better (Bringle, 2021).

<u>Fatigue</u>

A study conducted in 2017 indicated that acupuncture helped alleviate fatigue related to cancer as well as chronic fatigue. The practice can help improve your blood flow and decrease your blood pressure. This can decrease fatigue-inducing stress that affects your muscles, including your heart (Bringle, 2021).

<u>Vaginal dryness</u>

This uncomfortable condition is caused by hormone imbalances. When the acupuncture needles are inserted in specific points then neurochemicals are released which can help correct the imbalances (Bringle, 2021).

How to choose an acupuncturist

You want to make sure that your experience is safe and effective. It is imperative that you choose an acupuncturist who is an expert in their field. Not only do you want the acupuncturist to know how and where to place the needles, you also want to make sure that the needles are sterilized and the facilities are clean. The Mayo Clinic (2023) states that you would find an acupuncturist the same way that you would find any medical professional. You might start by asking friends or members of your support group for references. In addition, you can ask your regular doctor for a recommendation. You can also visit https://medicalacupuncture.org/find-an-acupuncturist/ to find a certified acupuncturist who is in your area.

Once you have found one, you can talk to the practitioners and ask them what your treatment would entail. You should ask how acupuncture will help mitigate your menopausal symptoms. In addition, you should also find out how much it costs and whether your insurance will cover it.

Breathing Exercises

Let's talk about breathing. I know that you are already doing that. However, you are likely breathing incorrectly. Most of us breathe shallowly, with our belly rising and falling when we inhale and then exhale. The correct way to breathe is to inhale deeply and then exhale completely. Breathing correctly can help us deal with our menopausal symptoms better. There are also specific breathing exercises that you can do to help mitigate those symptoms.

According to Providence (2021), our heart beats faster, and we breathe more quickly when we are stressed out. However, we can calm our heart rates and our minds when we take longer, deeper breaths. By taking fuller breaths, we are also able to improve our focus and our concentration.

The great thing about breathing exercises is that you can do them at any time and any place. As soon as you start to feel stressed out or you feel a hot flash coming on, you can start practicing one of the techniques.

<u>Deep Breathing</u>

Deep breathing is a great way to handle stress. When you are in a stressful situation, your heart rate increases, and your blood pressure increases. Unfortunately, when you suffer from chronic stress, it can lead to heart disease and weight gain, both of which are unfortunate byproducts of menopause. Like all techniques, the more you practice, the better you will become. Think about setting aside some time in the morning and in the evening before you are ready for bed to help you relax. Bolen (2020) describes the steps entailed with deep breathing.

1. Sit, with your back straight, in a chair. Both feet should be flat on the floor.

2. Put one of your hands on your stomach. Your pinky finger should be just above your navel.

3. Focus on how your belly rises and falls with your breathing. You can feel your diaphragm, which is the muscle that you use to breathe.

4. Observe how your belly feels like a balloon filling up as you inhale and then deflating as you exhale.

5. Your other hand should be on your chest. Keep the hand still so that your diaphragm is doing all the work. Your shoulders should also be relaxed. They should not move as you breathe.

6. Inhale as you slowly count to three.

7. Exhale as you slowly count to three. Think of the word "relax" as the air flows out of you. Saying this word to yourself each time will eventually make it a cue that is associated with relaxing. This means that you will think the word once you practice enough, and your body will automatically know to relax.

8. Keep your focus on your diaphragm, noticing how your hand moves out when you inhale and moves in as you exhale.

Bolen (2020) reminds you not to hold your breath after you inhale or exhale. She says that eventually, once you practice deep breathing, you will be able to lengthen your breaths.

<u>Boxed or square breathing</u>

Another breathing technique that you can use to help control your hot flashes, high blood pressure, fatigue, anxiety, or other symptoms of menopause is boxed breathing. Like deep breathing, you can practice this technique anywhere and anytime. Jones (2022) describes the technique:

1. Inhale through your nose to the count of four.

2. Hold the air in for the count of four.

3. Exhale through your mouth to the count of four.

4. Hold your breath out to the count of four.

Jones (2022) suggests you visualize a square while repeating this technique as often as possible.

<u>4-7-8 breathing technique</u>

In addition to the other benefits, this breathing technique can help you fight your cravings for food, help fight insomnia, and help you manage your emotional responses. It helps decrease your cortisol levels. Jones (2022) explains the steps of this technique:

1. Inhale through your nose to the count of four.

2. Hold the air in to the count of seven.

3. Exhale through your mouth to the count of eight.

<u>Paced breathing</u>

This breathing technique has you focus on taking controlled deep breaths that help slow your breathing. You will focus on your diaphragm as you engage in paced breathing (Jones, 2020).

1. Inhale for five seconds. Feel your chest expand as you breathe.

2. Exhale for five seconds.

3. Practice paced breathing for at least fifteen minutes

each day. You should use the paced breathing technique when you feel a hot flash starting.

<u>Word repetition</u>

Word repetition breathing can help you focus your attention away from your anxieties and help you relax, even during the discomfort of hot flashes. Jones (2020) describes the steps.

1. Choose a word to focus on.

2. Breath naturally.

3. Silently repeat your word as you exhale.

4. Practice this ten to twenty minutes daily.

<u>Autogenic training</u>

Jones (2020) states that lacking positive thoughts can be harmful. Use positive affirmations to achieve a better frame of mind.

1. Find a quiet spot to sit comfortably.

2. Practice deep breathing while you repeat affirmations. Examples that Jones (2020) gives are "I am calm, healthy, whole, and complete," "I choose joy and peace," and "I let go of things I cannot control."

There are many benefits of breathing exercises regardless of the breathing technique that you choose to use. The best thing about them is that you can practice them any time you start to feel a hot flash coming on or you start to feel stressed out and anxious.

Exercise

Exercising can help you deal with the symptoms of menopause. One reason is that women tend to gain abdominal fat when they go through menopause. Exercising on a regular basis can help decrease fat. In addition, staying at a healthy weight can help decrease your risks of heart disease and type 2 diabetes. It can also help lessen the risks of some types of cancer, such as breast, endometrial, and colon cancers. Exercise can also slow the rate of bone loss. In addition, exercises cause your brain to release feel-good hormones, such as endorphins, which decrease your risk of depression, stress, and anxiety. In addition, exercise can help slow the decline in cognitive functions (Mayo Clinic, 2023).

Exercises to do

According to the Mayo Clinic (2023), you should be engaged in moderate aerobic exercises for at least a hundred and fifty minutes weekly or vigorous aerobic activity for at least seventy-five minutes each week. You should also try strength training twice a week. The Mayo Clinic (2023) suggests that you consider the following type of exercise:

<u>Aerobic (cardio) activity:</u> Aerobics can help you lose extra pounds and stay at a healthy weight. Cohen (2022) states that cardio activity reduces your risk of heart disease and helps you clear your mind. It helps to improve your sleep and mood. You can engage in many aerobic exercises, such as swimming, jogging, brisk walking, or biking.

<u>Strength (weight) training:</u> Regular strength training can help you lose inches, burn off calories, and strengthen your muscles. It helps to improve your joint health and to decrease potential musculoskeletal problems later on. You can choose hand-held weights or machines. Mayo Clinic

(2023) recommends that you "Choose a weight or resistance level heavy enough to tire your muscles after about 12 repetitions." As you become stronger, you can gradually increase the weight or resistance levels.

<u>High-impact exercise:</u> According to Cohen (2023), the best way to prevent osteoporosis and fractures is to engage in high-impact exercises, as it helps to build up the bones when they are working against gravity. "Bone is stimulated through impact – particularly when you're changing directions, turning side to side, or making quick changes." Hiking, tennis, and soccer are some activities that qualify as high-impact exercises.

<u>Stretching:</u> Stretching your muscles helps to improve flexibility. Take the time to stretch after each workout because that is when your muscles are most receptive to stretching.

<u>Stability and balance:</u> Improving your balance helps to improve your stability. Improved stability can help reduce your risk of falls. You should try simple balancing activities such as brushing your hair while you are standing on one leg. Tai chi is also recommended to help improve your balance.

Keep motivated

There are so many things that I *want* to do, but I don't have the motivation to do them. Exercising is one. Therefore, I use different strategies, as described by the Mayo Clinic (2023) to help me get started.

1. Set realistic goals – SMART goals. These are goals

that are specific, measurable, achievable, relevant and time-bound. Instead of merely saying that I'm going to exercise today, I would say that I will walk briskly for twenty minutes after dinner.

2. Update your goals as you continue to grow. This month I might walk briskly for twenty minutes after dinner. Then, once I'm able to achieve that goal easily, I might add some minutes to that goal or even add in twelve sets of strength training exercises.

3. Team up with a person. It's harder to back out of an exercise regimen if you are accountable to another person.

4. Keep a journal of your successes. Once you achieve something positive, it motivates you to keep working.

Kegel Exercises

I will admit that sometimes I have been the person who might tinkle a little when I sneeze. Incontinence is one of the unfortunate symptoms associated with menopause. Doing kegel exercises will strengthen the muscles that support the bladder, bowel, and vagina. You can do them anywhere. These exercises help improve your flexibility, strength, coordination, and blood flow. Mayo Clinic (2023) describes how to do these exercises.

1. The first step is to find the right muscles by stopping the urination midstream. The muscle that you are using is what you will be strengthening. You can do the exercises in any position.

2. To do the exercise, Mayo Clinic (2023) suggests that you

pretend to sit on a marble and then tighten your pelvic muscles as though you are trying to lift the marble. Hold the muscles tight for three seconds, then release them for three seconds.

3. you must be only tightening your pelvic muscles during this exercise. Ensure you are not tightening other muscles, such as your abs. Make sure that you breathe while your muscles are tight – breathe normally.

4. Repeat the exercises at least three times a day. You should do three sets of ten to fifteen reps.

5. Don't practice tightening your muscles when urinating because it might make your bladder not emptier completely.

Tai Chi

Tai Chi is considered to be a form of both meditation and exercise and is referred to as "meditation in motion." However, because it is so healthy, Harvard Medical School (2022) said it should be called "medicine in motion." The National Center for Complementary and Integrative Health said, "mind and body practices such as yoga, tai chi, qigong, and acupuncture may help reduce the severity of menopausal symptoms, including the frequency and intensity of hot flashes, sleep and mood disturbances, stress, and muscle and joint pain," (Omega, 2023). A comprehensive review conducted by the *American Journal of Health Promotion* indicates there are a lot of benefits of tai chi, including relief from menopausal symptoms. Studies done by Harvard Medical School also indicated that tai chi is a safe, effective way to help menopausal women to maintain bone density (Omega, 2023).

There are a lot of other benefits of tai chi. One is that it can help you develop upper and lower body strength. Harvard Medical School (2022) says that if you practice tai chi regularly, it can be compared to resistance training and brisk walks. It can also help you become more flexible. Some studies have indicated that tai chi can help you improve your balance and decrease falls. It can also provide some aerobic benefits depending on the forms.

Tai chi is a low-impact exercise. You will go through a series of motions slowly, without pausing. While you are going through the movements, you will make sure that you focus on your breathing and on your physical sensations. Tai chi has many differences from standard exercises, according to Harvard Medical School (2022). While practicing tai chi, your movements are not as forced as they are in regular exercises. Unlike regular exercises, the movements are circular. Another difference is that our muscles are relaxed when we practice tai chi, not tense. You do not fully extend or bend your joints nor do you stretch your connective tissues. Tai chi is adaptive, and most people, even those who use a wheelchair or who have other disabilities, can perform this exercise. No special equipment is needed.

Get started

Harvard Medical School (2022) discusses several considerations when you are thinking about getting started with tai chi.

Don't let the language intimidate you. Some people might be intimidated by the names of different branches of tai chi. The names, such as Yang, Wu, and Cheng, were given to those who developed different forms. Some of these forms focus on the martial arts facets, while other forms emphasize healing and stress reduction. Some of the forms involve longer movement sequences, while others are shorter and emphasize breathing and meditation. It is more important that you consider which forms will help you mitigate your menopausal symptoms than worry about what they are called.

Consult your doctor. If you have some medical conditions, such as musculoskeletal, or if you take medication that might make you dizzy or lightheaded, then you should talk to your doctor before starting tai chi. However, Harvard Medical School (2022) states that it is so safe that your doctor would tell you to give it a go.

Think about observing and taking a class. The easiest way to learn tai chi is for you to observe a class. You can watch the teacher leading the class, receive feedback from the instructor, and experience group support. Most teachers will allow you to watch a class to make sure that you are comfortable with how the classes are taught. You can also find a teacher who will work with you on an individual basis. The local Y, community center, or senior center might be able to point you in the right direction. You can also check out the link: https://taichiforhealthinstitute.org/instructors/ to search for board-certified instructors in your area.

If you prefer to learn and practice at your home, then you can rent a video or watch one online. There are books about tai chi, but Harvard Medical School (2022) states that it might be difficult to understand the flow of the movements from pictures.

Talk to the instructor. If you choose to work with an instructor, you must talk to the person to ensure they will make a good fit. Because instructors don't have to be certified, you will want to ask for references. You also need to make sure that the instructor will consider your health needs and your coordination and fitness levels.

Dress comfortably. Your clothes should be loose fitting and not restrict your movements. You can either perform tai chi barefoot or wear lightweight, flexible shoes. The shoes shouldn't slip and help you balance. The soles should have thin soles so that you can feel the ground. Harvard Medical School (2022) said that running shoes are not suitable, because they are designed to push you forward.

Monitor your progress. Harvard Medical School (2022) states that most programs that were researched lasted a minimum of twelve weeks, which included instruction one or two days a week and home practice. At the end of a twelve-week period, you can determine whether you enjoy practicing tai chi and whether you have experienced any changes in your physical or psychological well-being.

How it's done

You start off a tai chi class by doing warm-up exercises that include easy movements, such as shoulder circles, turning your head from one side to the other, and rocking back and forth. These movements can help loosen up the joints and muscles and help you focus on your bodily sensations and breathing (Harvard Medical School, 2022).

Instruction and practice of tai chi forms come after the warm-ups. Forms are movement sets. Short forms might include twelve or fewer movements, whereas long forms might include hundreds of movements. The type of style will dictate whether you are using large or small movements. If you are a beginner or not in good condition, a short form with smaller and slower movements would likely be recommended (Harvard Medical School, 2022).

Qigong or chi kung means "breath work" or "energy work" (Harvard Medical School, 2022). This part of the class consists of gentle breathing that is sometimes combined with movement. The point of this part of the exercise is to help relax your mind and to mobilize your energy. Qigong can be done whether you are sitting down, standing up, or lying down (Harvard Medical School, 2022).

Turn Your Radio On

Think about the last time that you were doing some chores and you had music playing. Chances are you had a better attitude toward your tasks, you were more upbeat, you were moving faster and you accomplished your tasks a lot more quickly than you would have if you were working in silence.

Listening to music can decrease anxiety and depression. Music helps decrease your cortisol levels, which increases your blood pressure and your risk of heart disease. This can lead to the ability to sleep better at night and decrease certain health issues, such as heart disease. As an added benefit, your serotonin and endorphin levels increase which helps to improve your mood. (Providence, 2021)

There have been a lot of different studies that have proven that music can improve your physical health. According to a study done by the American College of Cardiology that tracked patients who already had a heart attck, listening to music for thirty minutes each day decreased their risk of heart failure by eighteen percent, decreased risk of heart attacks by twenty percent, decreased the need for bypass surgery by twenty percent, and decreased the rate of death from cardiac arrest by sixteen percent (Napoli, 2020).

Other Relaxation Methods

There are many other ways that you can relax to improve your health, your sleeping, and your mood.

1. Take a walk
2. Engage in a hobby
3. Take some time just for you
4. Aroma therapy
5. Draw
6. Write in a journal
7. Get a massage
8. Take a warm bath
9. Play with your pet
10. Read a book

. . .

Conclusion

Now you have accumulated a lot of tools that can help you handle the symptoms that came barging into your life with perimenopause and menopause. Not all of them will be your cup of tea. You have to decide what will work for you. Take a moment and write down three methods that you can use to help you overcome the symptoms of menopause. Then, continue on to the next chapter of questions and answers.

Chapter 7

Questions and Answers

Following are some questions and answers about menopause women might have (University of Iowa, 2022).

Q: What are the symptoms of perimenopause and menopause?

A: Women may experience different symptoms with different frequencies and severity. Some symptoms are hot flashes, night sweats, mood swings, insomnia, joint pain, vaginal dryness, forgetfulness, and weight gain.

Q: Why do menopausal symptoms occur?

A: They occur because women's estrogen levels tend to

decrease through menopause. The decrease in estrogen can have many effects – not only the obvious ones – but also an increased risk of heart disease, osteoporosis, type 2 diabetes, and some types of cancer.

Q: Will I go through menopause if I have a hysterectomy?

A: If you have a partial hysterectomy and your uterus is taken, but your ovaries remain, then you will not go through menopause right away. This is because estrogen is mostly produced in your ovaries. A partial hysterectomy means you will be unable to get pregnant and will not menstruate. If your ovaries are removed then you will go into menopause.

Q: Do women have sexual problems during and after menopause?

A: Women can experience sexual problems, including a lack of arousal, pain during sex, a loss of interest, and the ability to orgasm. Talk to your doctor if you are experiencing any of these issues.

Q: Why is forgetfulness an issue during menopause?

A: Many women state that they have cognitive changes once they reach perimenopause and menopause. This is often due to a lack of sleep and fatigue. Try to get enough rest and stay active. However, if forgetfulness still has a negative impact on your life, talk to your doctor.

Dr. Shana Miles (2020) also discusses some commonly asked questions women have about menopause.

Q: Should I do hormone replacement therapy?

A: Hormone therapy is an option to help you deal with the symptoms of menopause. However, before you start HRT, try some other options, such as exercising, meditation, etc.

Q: Should I use supplements?

A: Be very careful about using supplements. Because the FDA does not regulate them, you don't know what levels of the different hormones you are getting. You also don't know what extra ingredients are added. Talk to your doctor before deciding on any supplements.

Q: Do I still need to have the annual visit?

A: Absolutely. There is still a risk of uterine, endometrial, and ovarian cancer during and after menopause. Your doctor will also check for STDs. It will also allow you to discuss incontinence, sex, and other issues.

. . .

Q: What about pap tests and mammograms?

A: You should continue to get pap tests until you are at least sixty-five and mammograms until you are at least seventy-five. Your doctor will talk to you about getting them longer if you have a higher risk.

Prologue

"If you are facing in the right direction, all you need to do is keep on walking." ~ Buddha

Perimenopause and menopause can be an exciting transitional time in our lives. Some women, like myself, don't even know that they are going through perimenopause at first. The symptoms sneak up on them like ninjas. For other women, the symptoms explode into their lives like a hurricane.

Regardless of how you enter this phase in your life, it doesn't have to be that scary time in your life that signifies that you are getting "old." As a matter of fact, the opposite is true. You've taken the first step in staying your normal, young, happy self – you educated yourself.

The first step is learning about your body and what it is

going through. You now know that the decrease in estrogen can cause your body to feel as though it is going to combust into flames one minute and feel like it is in the arctic the next minute. Sleep is elusive; you forget things, and let's not even talk about those mood swings.

Luckily, there are a lot of methods and techniques that you can use to help decrease the frequency and intensity of your symptoms.

One of the most common complaints is hot flashes. You can deal with them by carrying around a personal fan. Dress in layers of loose-fitting clothes. Use cool images, yoga, meditation, and mindfulness to help you overcome the severity. You should also avoid spicy food, alcohol, and caffeine.

Insomnia is another complaint. Not only is insomnia a miserable experience, but it also contributes to high blood pressure, mood swings, irritability, fatigue, and forgetfulness. Sleep hygiene is a great way to help you beat insomnia. Exercising, breathing exercises, yoga, and meditation are other methods you can engage in to help you get some rest. You can also indulge in foods that will help you get a good night's rest.

Many of the same techniques that will help you over-come your hot flashes and insomnia will, at the same time, help to mitigate the other symptoms of menopause. Eating right, exercising, and other techniques will help reduce blood pressure and the risks of heart disease, osteoporosis, type 2 diabetes, and some types of cancer.

It is important to remember that menopause doesn't own you, and it doesn't get to dictate your life. By reading this book you have put a number of tools in your toolbox that will let you control the severity and intensity of the symptoms and help you to continue living a happy, healthy life.

I hope you enjoyed this book. If you did, please leave a review. Cheers.

Bibliography

Abramson, A. (November 1, 2022). *Meditation Techniques to Help with Menopause Symptoms*. Stripes. https://iamstripes.com/blogs/mental-health/meditation-techniques-to-help-with-menopause-symptoms

Alloy Staff. (November 9, 2022). *What Causes Late-Onset Menopause*. https://www.myalloy.com/blog/late-onset-menopause

Babuata, L. (N.D.). *Meditation for Beginners: 20 Practical Tips for Understanding the Mind*. Zen Mind. https://zenhabits.net/meditation-guide/.

Belcher, N, Ph.D. (2023). *Why Progesterone-Only*. Winona https://bywinona.com/journal/why-progesterone-only

Bolen, B. (January 28, 2020). *How to Do Breathing Exercises*. Very Well Health. https://www.verywellhealth.com/how-to-do-deep-breathing-exercises-1945350

Bringle, J. (May 26, 2021). *6 Symptoms of Menopause Acupuncture Might Help*. Healthline. https://www.healthline.com/health/menopause/acupuncture-for-menopause-how-this-alternative-therapy-brought-me-relief

Brown, M.J. (March 29, 2022). *11 Natural Ways to Reduce Symptoms of Menopause*. Healthline. https://www.healthline.com/nutrition/11-natural-menopause-tips

Burnett, T. MD. (2023). *Bioidentical Hormones: Are They Safe?* https://www.mayoclinic.org/diseases-conditions/menopause/expert-answers/bioidentical-hormones/faq-20058460?p=1

National Cancer Insitute. (2023). *Menopausal Hormone Therapy and Cancer*. https://www.cancer.gov/about-cancer/causes-prevention/risk/hormones/mht-fact-sheet

Cleveland Health Clinic. (2023). *Bioidentical Hormones*. https://my.clevelandclinic.org/health/articles/15660-bioidentical-hormones

Cleveland Health Clinic. (2023). *Menopause: What It Is, Age, Stages, Signs, & Side Effects*. https://my.clevelandclinic.org/health/diseases/21841-menopause

Cleveland Health Clinic. (2023). *Therapy for Menopause: Types, Benefits, and Risks.* https://my.clevelandclinic.org/health/treatments/15245-hormone-therapy-for-menopause-symptoms

Cohen, M. (July 26, 2022). *7 Best Exercises to Do During Menopause, According to Experts.* Retrieved from https://www.goodhousekeeping.com/health/fitness/g40476189/menopause-exercises/?utm_source=google&utm_medium=cpc&utm_campaign=arb_ga_ghk_d_b m_prog_org_us_g40476189&gclid= CjwKCAjw_MqgBhAGEiwAnYOAerwxX6OxHUl_y5up s4kk1WUQ47CqfsEcDUUWhXnqvrMYQQ8686tmfhoCVDIQAv D_BwE

Currie, H. Dr. (September 2021). *Menopause and Insomnia.* https://www.womens-health-concern.org/wp-content/uploads/2022/12/17-WHC-FACTSHEET-Menopause-and-insomnia-NOV2022-B.pdf

Durward, E. (January 25, 2021). *Relaxation tips to help ease menopause symptoms.* A. Vogel. https://www.avogel.co.uk/health/menopause/videos/relaxation-tips-to-help-ease-menopause-symptoms/

Elliott, B. R.D. (February 22, 2023). *The 9 Best Foods and Drinks to Have Before Bed.* Healthline https://www.healthline.com/nutrition/9-foods-to-help-you-sleep

Everyday Yoga. (April 12, 2015). *How to Do Reclined Bound Angle Pose in Yoga.* https://www.everydayyoga.com/blogs/guides/how-to-do-reclined-bound-angle-pose-in-yoga

Everheart, D. (2023). *Guided Meditation: Help for Anxiety, Stress, Sleep, and More.* The Art of Living. https://www.artofliving.org/us-en/meditation/beginners-guide/online-guided-meditation#author-description

Faris, S. (February 13, 2017). *Late-Onset Menopause: What is Causing Your Delay?* Healthline. https://www.healthline.com/health/menopause/late-onset

Gennev. (2023). *10 Red Flag Warning Signs of Menopause.* https://www.gennev.com/education/warning-signs-of-menopause.

Goodreads. (2023). *59 Quotes.* https://www.goodreads.com/quotes/tag/menopause

Groves, M. (November 23, 2018). *Diet: How What You Eat Affects Your Symptoms. Healthline.* https://www.healthline.com/nutrition/menopause-diet

Gura, T. (January 15, 2019). *Yoga for Menopause: How to Relieve Common Symptoms.* Yoga Journal. https://www.yogajournal.com/lifestyle/health/womens-health/yoga-for-menopause-relieve-common-symptoms/

Harvard Medical School. (May 24, 2022). *The Health Benefits of Tai Chi.* https://www.health.harvard.edu/staying-healthy/the-health-benefits-of-tai-chi

Higuera, V. (November 23, 2023). *Happy Baby Pose: How to Do, Benefits, and History.* Healthline. https://www.healthline.com/health/happy-baby-pose

Howshaw, C. (March 29, 2022). *What is Mindfulness: Benefits, How to Practice, and More.* https://www.healthline.com/health/mind-body/what-is-mindfulness

Hunter, M. & Smith, M., Dr. (2023). *Cognitive Behavioural Therapy for Menopausal Women.* Women's Health Concern. https://www.womens-health-concern.org/wp-content/uploads/2023/02/02-WHC-FACT SHEET-CBT-WOMEN-FEB-2023-A.pdf

Jack, C. (May 24, 2020). *Can Hypnotherapy Help Me During Menopause?* Psychology Today. https://www.psychologytoday.com/us/blog/women-autism-spectrum-disorder/202005/can-hypnotherapy-help-me-during-menopause

John Hopkins Health. (2023). *Acupuncture.* https://www.hopkinsmedicine.org/health/wellness-and-prevention/acupuncture

John Hopkins Health. (2023). *Estrogen's Effect on the Female Body.* https://www.hopkinsmedicine.org/health/conditions-and-diseases/estrogens-effects-on-the-female-body

John Hopkins Health. (2023). *Perimenopause.* https://www.hopkinsmedicine.org/health/conditions-and-diseases/perimenopause

Jones, B. (April 12, 2022). *Late-Onset Menopause: Causes, Age, Risk Factors.* Very Well Health. https://www.verywellhealth.com/late-menopause-5219757

Jones, B. (April 11, 2022). *Ways to Relax During Menopause.* Very Well Health. https://www.verywellhealth.com/menopause-relaxation-techniques-5219886

Mayo Clinic. (2023). *Acupuncture.* https://www.mayoclinic.org/tests-procedures/acupuncture/about/pac-20392763

Mayo Clinic. (2023). *Fitness Tips for Menopause: Why Fitness Counts.* https://www.mayoclinic.org/healthy-lifestyle/womens-health/in-depth/fitness-tips-for-menopause/art-20044602

Mayo Clinic. (2023). *Hormone Therapy: Is It Right for You?* https://www.mayoclinic.org/diseases-conditions/menopause/in-depth/hormone-therapy/art-20046372

Mayo Clinic. (2023). *Kegel Exercises: A how-to guide for women.* https://www.mayoclinic.org/healthy-lifestyle/womens-health/in-depth/kegel-exercises/art-20045283

Mayo Clinic. (2023). *Menopause.* https://www.mayoclinic.org/diseases-conditions/menopause/diagnosis-treatment/drc-20353401

Mayo Clinic. (2019, January 17). *Mindfulness May Ease Menopausal Symptoms. ScienceDaily.* March 11, 2023 from www.sciencedaily.com/releases/2019/01/190117090449.htm

Mayo Clinic. (2023). *Perimenopause.* https://www.mayoclinic.org/diseases-conditions/perimenopause/symptoms-causes/syc-20354666

Mayo Clinic. (2023). *Perimenopause.* https://www.mayoclinic.org/diseases-conditions/perimenopause/diagnosis-treatment/drc-20354671

Medline Plus. (2023). *Progesterone.* https://medlineplus.gov/druginfo/meds/a604017.html

Miles, S. M.D. (October 2020). *5 of the Most Common Questions About Menopause.* The American College of Obstetricians and Gynecologists. https://www.acog.org/womens-health/experts-and-stories/the-latest/5-of-the-most-common-questions-about-menopause

Napoli, N. (March 18, 2020). *Music as Medicine? 30 Minutes a Day Shows Benefits After Heart Attack.* American College of Cardiology. https://www.acc.org/about-acc/press-releases/2020/03/18/09/02/music-as-medicine-30-minutes-a-day-shows-benefits-after-heart-attack.

National Health Services. (2023). *Hormone Replacement Therapy.* https://www.nhs.uk/conditions/hormone-replacement-therapy-hrt/

National Institute on Aging. (2023). *Hot Flashes: What Can I Do?* https://www.nia.nih.gov/health/hot-flashes-what-can-i-do

National Institute on Aging. (2023). *Sex and Vaginal Dryness.* https://www.nia.nih.gov/health/sex-and-menopause-treatment-symptoms

National Institute on Aging. (2023). *What is Menopause?* https://www.nia.nih.gov/health/what-menopause

National Institute of Diabetes and Digestive and Kidney Diseases. (2023). *Bladder Infection.* https://www.niddk.nih.gov/health-information/urologic-diseases/bladder-infection-uti-in-adults

National Institute of Health. (2020). *Black Cohosh.* https://www.nccih.nih.gov/health/black-cohosh

Omega. (2023). *Managing Menopause with Qigong.* Retrieved from https://www.eomega.org/article/managing-menopause-with-qigong

Overall Motivation. (2023). *38 Menopause Quotes on Success in Life.* https://www.overallmotivation.com/quotes/menopause-quotes/

Pajer, N. (December 2, 2022). *50 Best Meditation Quotes: Short, Inspirational Quotes About Meditation.* Parade: Entertainment, Recipes, Health, Life, Holidays. https://parade.com/1066461/nicolepajer/meditation-quotes/

Piedmont Atlanta Fitness Center. (2023). *How Exercise Helps Balance Hormones.* https://www.piedmont.org/living-better/how-exercise-helps-balance-hormones

Pizer, A. (March 27, 2020). *How to Do Child's Pose (Balasana).* Very Well Fit. https://www.verywellfit.com/childs-pose-balasana-3567066

Pizer, A. (October 15, 2022). *How to do Corpse Pose (Savasana).* Very Well Fit. https://www.verywellfit.com/corpse-pose-savasana-3567112

Pizer, A. (July 16, 2021). *How to Do Downward Facing Dog (Adho Mukha Svanasana).* Very Well Fit. https://www.verywellfit.com/downward-facing-dog-adho-mukha-svanasana-3567072

Pizer, A. (December 21, 2022). *How to Do Mountain Pose.* Very Well Fit. https://www.verywellfit.com/mountain-pose-tadasana-3567127

Pizer, A. (May 24, 2021). *How to Do Plow Pose.* Very Well Fit. https://www.verywellfit.com/plow-pose-halasana-3567105

Pizer, A. (November 10, 2020). *How to Do Raised Hands Pose.* Very Well Fit. https://www.verywellfit.com/raised-hands-pose-urdhva-hastasana-3567131

Pizer, A. (July 01, 2020). *How to Do Reclined Goddess Pose.* Very Well Fit. https://www.verywellfit.com/reclined-goddess-pose-supta-baddha-konasana-3567149

Pizer, A. (January 18, 2021). *How to Do Reclined Hero Pose (Supta Virasana) in Yoga.* Very Well Fit. https://www.verywellfit.com/reclined-hero-pose-supta-virasana-3567051

Pizer, A. (December 11, 2021). *How to Do Shoulderstand (Salamba Sarvangasana): Techniques, Benefits, Variations.* Very Well Fit. https://www.verywellfit.com/shoulderstand-salamba-sarvangasana-3567115

Pizer, A. (October 25, 2022). *How to Do Standing Forward Bend.* Very Well Health. https://www.verywellfit.com/standing-forward-bend-uttanasana-3567133

Providence. (March 7, 2021). *Meditation, Mindfulness, and Music for Heart Health. https://www.providence.org/news/uf/649404374*

Saranchock, C. (2023). *Progressive Muscle Relaxation Meditation.* Help Guide. https://www.helpguide.org/meditations/progressive-muscle-relaxation-meditation.htm

Scott, L. MD. (2023). *Progesterone Benefits.* https://www.leighannscottmd.com/progesterone-benefits/

Spritzler, F. (May 12, 2021). *How to Lose Weight Around Menopause (and Keep It Off).* Healthline. https://www.healthline.com/nutrition/lose-weight-in-menopause

Tewari, A. (2023). *Top 50 Wellness Quotes for a Healthier Life.* Gratitude Blog. https://blog.gratefulness.me/wellness-quotes/

University of Iowa. (May 23, 2022). *Menopause: Frequently Asked Questions. https://uihc.org/health-topics/menopause-frequently-asked-questions*

Vogel, K. (February 14, 2023). *50 Real Menopause Quotes.* Parade. https://parade.com/1239990/kaitlin-vogel/menopause-quotes/

WebMD. (2023). *Hormone Replacement Therapy Types and Side Effects.* https://www.webmd.com/menopause/menopause-hormone-therapy

WebMD. (June 8, 2021). *Relaxation Techniques During Menopause: Breathing, Music, and More. https://www.webmd.com/menopause/guide/learning-relax-during-menopause*

WebMD. (September 13, 2006). *Meditation May Cool Hot Flashes. https://www.webmd.com/menopause/news/20060913/meditation-may-cool-hot-flashes*

White, A. & Cherney, K. (July 10, 2021). *Phytoestrogens: Benefits, Menopause, Side Effects, and Food.* Healthline. https://www.healthline.com/health/phytoestrogens

Bibliography

Yoga Basics. (2023). *Wide-Legged Forward Bend Pose (Prasarita Padottanasana) * Yoga Basics. https://www.yogabasics.com/asana/wide-legged-forward-bend/*

141

www.ingramcontent.com/pod-product-compliance
Lightning Source LLC
Chambersburg PA
CBHW051307250726
48656CB00004B/1526